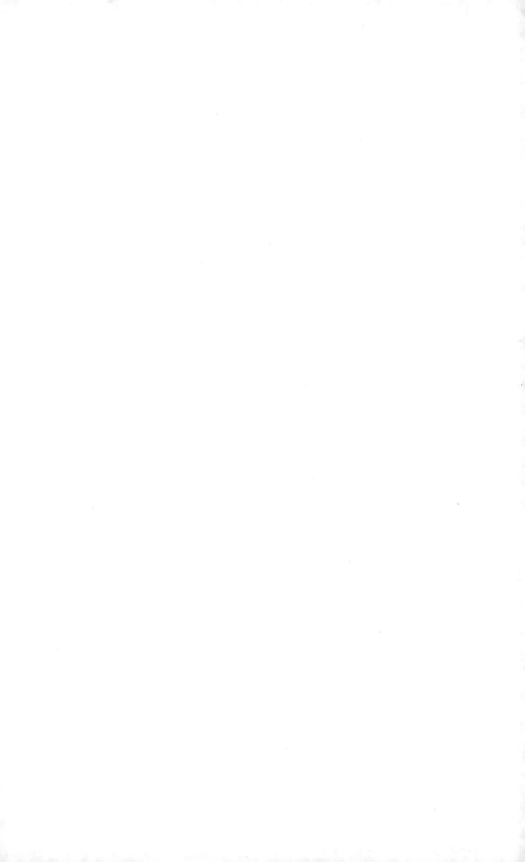

▷ Using research for effective health promotion

▷ **Using research for effective health promotion**

Edited by
Sandy Oliver and Greet Peersman

Open University Press
Buckingham · Philadelphia

Open University Press
Celtic Court
22 Ballmoor
Buckingham
MK18 1XW

email: enquiries@openup.co.uk
world wide web: www.openup.co.uk

and
325 Chestnut Street
Philadelphia, PA 19106, USA

First Published 2001

A catalogue record of this book is available from the British Library

ISBN   0 335 20870 3 (pb)   0 335 20871 1 (hb)

Library of Congress Cataloging-in-Publication Data
Using research for effective health promotion / edited by Sandy Oliver and
Greet Peersman.
     p. cm.
   Includes bibliographical references and index.
   ISBN 0-335-20871-1 (hbk.) – ISBN 0-335-20870-3 (pbk.)
     1. Health promotion. 2. Health promotion–Research. 3. Primary care
(Medicine) 4. Evidence-based medicine. I. Oliver, Sandy, 1955–
II. Peersman, Greet.
RA427.8.U84   2001
613–dc21   00-065245

Typeset by Graphicraft Limited, Hong Kong
Printed in Great Britain by Biddles Limited, Guildford and King's Lynn

▷ Contents

▷ Notes on contributors

Simon Forrest is a Research Fellow in the Department of Sexually Transmitted Diseases at University College London. He is working on a collaborative study with the Social Science Research Unit at the Institute of Education into peer-led sex education in secondary schools in England (the RIPPLE study). His background is in health-related research and health promotion with young people, and he has contributed to books and papers and resources for young people and teachers on sex, sexuality and health.

Angela Harden is currently undertaking research within two programmes of work at the EPPI-Centre which aim to facilitate the use of research evidence to inform policy and practice in health promotion and education. She is particularly interested in the challenges involved in understanding the contributions of different types of research to policy and practice. Her previous work has included primary research examining the provision of sexual health services for young people.

Amanda Nicholas developed and now maintains the information management systems at the EPPI-Centre. She runs the enquiry service about evidence-based health promotion. She is now developing systems to support people collaborating with the EPPI-Centre in preparing systematic reviews in education. She is practically involved in promoting health on a daily basis as a competitive salsa dancing teacher.

Ann Oakley is Professor of Sociology and Social Policy and Director of the Social Science Research Unit at the University of London Institute of Education. She has many years' experience of social science research, and has published many books on gender, the family and women's health. Her recent interests focus on the role and methodology of social interventions.

Sandy Oliver works within the EPPI-Centre to further evidence-informed education and health promotion. She is particularly interested in developing ways to enable service users to influence what research is undertaken, and how. Her interest in research for policy and practice was stimulated by her experience of using maternity services and as an antenatal teacher and member of the Research and Information Group of the National Childbirth Trust.

Greet Peersman has been involved in the establishment and running of the EPPI-Centre from 1995 until 1999, and is now a Visiting Fellow. She is currently working at the US Centers for Disease Control and Prevention, where she is involved in systematically reviewing the effectiveness of HIV prevention, and in monitoring and evaluation of an extensive HIV prevention and care programme in Africa and Asia. She is also an editor for the Cochrane HIV/AIDS Group. Greet previously worked in health education in Zimbabwe and as a health researcher at the University of Antwerp in Belgium.

Vicki Strange is currently working on the RIPPLE trial: a randomized controlled trial of pupil peer-led sex education in schools. She is also undertaking doctoral research examining the utility of using randomized controlled trials for evaluating social interventions. Before joining the SSRU in 1997 she worked for Waltham Forest Education Authority, managing a team who provided supported employment services for adults with learning difficulties.

James Thomas has been with the EPPI-Centre since it was established in 1995. He has been responsible for the development of information systems to facilitate the production and dissemination of systematic reviews. Also employed with funding from the Department for Education and Employment to adapt EPPI-Centre tools for the field of education.

▷ Acknowledgements

Ideas presented in this book have evolved through the authors' direct experience of research and through discussions with people who have a special interest in the role of research in health promotion. It is often difficult to judge exactly when, how and under whose influence particular ideas crystallized, were better understood or better explained. We are grateful to many practitioners, policy makers and researchers who have engaged us in discussions about health promotion and the evidence available or needed to direct its further development. They have motivated us to reflect carefully on our work in the light of others' and the principles held by different people with an interest in this area.

In particular, we would like to acknowledge the influence and help of health promotion specialists who attended the 'Promoting Health After Sifting the Evidence' (PHASE) workshops in 1996 (see Chapter 11). Some of the book rests on work undertaken with colleagues. In particular, we are grateful to Chris Bonell for his historical analysis of health promotion and evidence-based policy and practice (Chapter 1); to Ros Weston for her work with us on the review of peer-delivered interventions (Chapters 8 and 9); and to Judith Lumley, Laura Oakley and Elizabeth Waters for their collaboration with us in work about qualitative data in systematic reviews of effectiveness (Chapter 12). We would like to thank Susan Charleston, who was involved in writing the first draft of Chapter 11, all the staff and students of the schools involved in the trial for their time, support and enthusiasm, the university students who enabled us to carry out the questionnaire survey in schools over the past two years and those who have provided secretarial support throughout the trial. We also particularly appreciate the stimulating discussions with other colleagues at the EPPI-Centre, particularly Rebecca Rees, Jonathan Shepherd and Ginny Brunton, and at the Social Science Research Unit and other research institutions, who continue to influence our work. We are indepted to Amanda Nicholas for her painstaking work in collating and checking the manuscript.

Much of this book is drawn from 'Field Co-ordination in Health Promotion Linked to the Cochrane Collaboration', a research project carried out by the Social Science Research Unit of the Institute of Education, University of London, with funding from the Department of Health. The views expressed are those of the authors and do not necessarily reflect those of the Department of Health or any other government department. Crown copyright material is reproduced by permission of the Controller of Her Majesty's Stationery Office.

▷ Preface

The backdrop for this book is the widely held conviction that health promotion can bring improved health and stem the spiralling costs of health care. Set against that is the growing concern about the evidence base for public policy generally, and the crisis of confidence this provokes for health promotion in particular, where the evidence of effectiveness is scant. The inherent value judgements of recognizing good health, and doubts about the comparative costs and benefits of preventive strategies and treatment, place health promotion under close scrutiny. These problems are being addressed on an international scale by systematic efforts to draw together the research evidence of the effects of health promotion, as well as other health interventions. This book describes the international endeavours of the Cochrane Collaboration for health care (see Chapter 1) and those evolving with the support of the World Wide Web for health promotion specifically (see Chapters 5 and 13).

Within this context, UK policies for managing and funding health promotion often affect the ways in which providers are able to improve their services (see Chapters 3 and 11). Health promotion providers are increasingly called on to justify investment in their services in terms of effectiveness, and to compete for continued funding, often as part of an annual cycle. Such pressures argue in favour of the increased use of interventions known to be effective, but in practice these pressures lead to reduced time available for evaluating new services or drawing on previous research reports for planning services. Thus a rift has appeared between practitioners exhorted to offer effective interventions, and researchers with the skills to supply some of the necessary information. This book bridges this rift by discussing the theoretical underpinning of health promotion and experimental methods in social science in an integrated framework; and by providing time-saving tools to draw on research quickly and critically.

In 1995, the Social Science Research Unit (SSRU) received a three-year grant from the Department of Health (DoH) to establish and coordinate an international effort aiming to advance evidence-based health promotion. This grant allowed for the continuation of a research programme on systematic reviews, and the establishment of an information, resource and training centre to promote the use of research in decision-making in health promotion. This centre was originally named the Centre for the Evaluation of Health Promotion and Social Interventions (EPI-Centre) and has since been renamed the Evidence-informed Policy and Practice Information and Coordinating Centre (EPPI-Centre). Recognition of the role of evidence in policy and practice decisions is spreading. The Department for Education and Employment (DfEE) has recently commissioned a parallel stream of work in which the EPPI-Centre supports groups of people who are systematically reviewing the research literature about interventions in education. A third stream of work reviews the literature about service user or 'consumer' involvement in research, which informs the systematic reviews in education and health promotion. In each stream of work the focus is on 'effectiveness'. This includes: what effective interventions are needed and are they acceptable, feasible and appropriate; how can effective interventions be developed; what interventions have proven to be effective, what have not and what seem promising; how and why are they effective (or not); in what (or whose) terms is effectiveness judged and how is it established?

Much of this book draws on the work that the EPPI-Centre team has undertaken since 1995, based on earlier work of the SSRU. It illustrates how our thinking and working practices have changed over time with the input from other researchers, policy makers and those delivering as well as those receiving health promotion services.

Over the past decades, health promotion has been struggling to establish itself as distinct from disease prevention, which is based on a medicalized notion of health and targets individual behaviour. Health promotion, on the other hand, strives to address the social, political and economic determinants of health seen as 'a complete state of physical, mental and social well-being', and to empower people to take charge of their own health. A lot of debate has therefore focused on what can really be called health promotion and how we know whether it works. Within this context the EPPI-Centre has taken the view that there is a wide range of interventions that *potentially* contribute to improving health, preventing disease and reducing disease impact and social inequalities. These interventions involve different sections of the public and different professionals; from health care workers addressing individual behaviour to politicians making policies on employment or housing conditions. In assessing the relative merits of such interventions, EPPI-Centre work has mainly focused on research on effectiveness, appropriateness and feasibility. As such, our work contributes to building the knowledge base of health promotion – including different types of research, as well as expert and lay opinion, that need to be considered when making informed decisions.

Work funded by the DoH grant has focused on a range of health promotion topics mainly relevant to young people; an initial concurrent three-year grant from the North Thames Regional Health Authority focused specifically on sexual health promotion, including HIV/AIDS prevention. Though we necessarily had to focus our work on some areas of health promotion, our methods and tools are designed to apply, with little or no adaptation, throughout the field.

The methods used by the EPPI-Centre have been adapted each time a new research question is tackled, building on new advances in systematic reviewing and taking into account criticism from end-users to previous review efforts. The work of the EPPI-Centre has been strongly influenced by methodological advances in systematically reviewing the effects of health care, which have been led primarily by those working in the field of medicine. Details of methods have been adapted to accommodate practical problems more often encountered in health promotion than in medicine: for instance, a sparsity of randomized controlled trials; interventions aimed at communities rather than individuals; and higher attrition rates with healthy populations in non-clinical settings. The ensuing reviews showed that it was possible to apply systematic methods to reviewing the effects of social interventions, even though these may differ appropriately in their detail from methods developed in medicine.

EPPI-Centre work has also focused on how the findings of an effectiveness review depend upon how it is done: for instance, how studies are sought and what criteria are used to include or exclude studies from the review. As with reviews in other areas of health care, major differences in the conclusions about effectiveness were found between systematic and non-systematic approaches to reviewing. Non-systematic approaches suggest that the vast majority of interventions are effective, and systematic approaches which draw on a wide range of study designs (including non-trials) also offer excessively promising conclusions. However, systematic reviews based on sound methodological criteria generated considerable controversy among health promotion practitioners, and were perceived as disregarding study designs other than trials in the development of health promotion services. More recent EPPI-Centre reviews have therefore tried to accommodate more of the concerns of practitioners, particularly: the lack of attention to the theoretical basis and implementation of interventions; varying 'quality' of interventions; and an interest in reviews focused primarily on interventions, settings or populations, rather than health problems. These efforts draw on the willingness to combine qualitative and quantitative, or observational and experimental, approaches, and a commitment to consumer involvement in research.

What to expect from this book

Health promotion can be seen as a subset of all social intervention, or it can be seen as part of the broader health services. In this book we take the view that lessons can be applied from both social science and health services research.

This book is rooted in the fundamental principles of both health promotion and evidence-informed policy and practice. This has implications for how appropriate research is undertaken and how it is used to inform services. The book focuses on the integration of evidence of feasibility, evidence of acceptability and evidence of effectiveness and, as such, aims to contribute to the cross-sectoral debate on how evidence-informed services could make a difference to users' health and satisfaction. It also provides practical tools to enable practitioners to apply their own judgement to research reports quickly and confidently, and describes new approaches to involving the public in evaluating health promotion services.

This book is of interest to all those wishing to contribute to the current movements towards effectiveness and consumer involvement in health services, including health promotion practitioners, service planners and lecturers and students of MSc and diploma courses in health promotion, public health, nursing, social work and voluntary services. In particular, health promotion practitioners may want to draw on it when: seeking to develop their understanding and critical use of research; preparing research-based service contracts; planning to strengthen their work with appropriate evaluation; preparing reports of their own work; or influencing the research agenda in health promotion. Funders may use it to be better aware of the opportunities and constraints for evidence-based health promotion when preparing contracts with service providers or researchers. Researchers may draw on the tools for identifying and reviewing research reports; for applying principles of integrating qualitative and experimental evaluation methods; and when considering practitioners and the public as co-directors of their work rather than just the subject of it. We hope that this book will also be a valuable tool for those who are targeted by health promotion research and practice; that it will increase their understanding and therefore their participation in setting the agenda, conducting the research and using the research findings.

The book is organized in four parts, each including a number of chapters. Some chapters provide the background and context of evidence-based health promotion; others present analyses of available research or offer tools to facilitate the use of research findings. Overall, the book is unique in describing and explaining advances in this field, and considering the relevance of research to service development and practice.

Part 1 has three chapters which are about theory and the need to ground health promotion in sound, methodologically diverse evidence. Chapter 1 addresses the theoretical underpinning of health promotion, its varying scope over time and its links with the social welfare field. It also discusses the position of health promotion within the move towards evidence-based health care. Chapter 2 looks at the origin of evaluation and describes the approaches that have been used to evaluate health promotion. It makes the argument for the integration of experimental and qualitative methods in developing evidence-based health promotion. In Chapter 3, the position of research in the decision-making process is discussed, and general ways of finding and classifying the widely dispersed research literature as a means to facilitating its use in service delivery are presented.

Part 2 provides in-depth discussion and practical tools to allow quick and critical use of research findings. Chapters 4 and 5 concentrate on how to find the evidence both quickly and comprehensively, including through accessing the World Wide Web. Once research reports are identified, there is a need for critically appraising the validity and usefulness of research findings, methods and tools for which are discussed in Chapter 6. Chapter 7 sets out how systematic reviews are undertaken and discusses the EPPI-Centre tools for analysing and integrating the findings from evaluation research in health promotion. It also signposts other sources of systematic reviews.

Part 3 takes young people's health as a case study, and illustrates how the issues discussed in Part 2 can be practically applied within both primary and secondary research. How studies can be integrated in a systematic review to answer questions of effectiveness, as well as questions of appropriateness, is presented in Chapter 8. Chapter 9 investigates the extent to which young people have been involved in health promotion studies and suggests ways for improving their participation. Ideally, primary research includes participation of the study population and integrates different research methods. Chapter 10 discusses the opportunities and challenges in trying to achieve that in a currently ongoing randomized controlled trial of school-based peer-led sex education.

Part 4 explains how health promotion and its evaluation is changing with political pressures, and presents the opportunities for health promotion to play an important role in the interrelated movements of evidence-based health and consumer involvement. It argues that the desire to meet the information needs of different end-users must influence the research process. Chapter 11 sets out how skills development is necessary but insufficient as a means for facilitating evidence-based health promotion and indicates that there is also a need to change the context in which health promotion is being provided. In Chapter 12 examples are presented of how 'consumers' can be involved in research and how they have influenced the nature of research and the degree to which it may be used. Finally, Chapter 13 describes the political influences of health promotion research and discusses the growing enthusiasm for experimental social research and a needs-led research agenda. It points to some important opportunities for better health in the future.

Evidence-based medicine has been led by medics, but evidence-based therapy, evidence-based nursing and evidence-based policy-making are increasingly attracting attention through journals and books. This book will lead the field in evidence-based health promotion and lay the foundation for evidence-informed education and public participation in research and policy development. These fields of interest deal with what are essentially social interventions, and overlap in their aim to educate and enable people to reach their full potential within the context of a conducive and supportive environment.

We have only just begun a long journey. Further advances will be recorded on the EPPI-Centre's Web site (http://eppi.ioe.ac.uk/). We invite readers to engage in a dialogue with us and with their colleagues and friends to further, and to improve upon, the knowledge-base of health promotion.

Sandy Oliver and Greet Peersman

▶ **Part I**

▷ Theory of health promotion and evaluation

▶ **1**

▷ # Promoting health: principles of practice and evaluation

▷ ## Greet Peersman

What does promoting health entail?

Public health has been defined as 'an organized response to the protection and promotion of human health which encompasses a concern with the environment, disease control, the provision of health care, health education and health promotion' (Research Unit in Health and Behavioural Change 1995: xvii). An ageing population, rising health care costs, a widening social class gradient in health and pressure from health lobby groups have put public health firmly on the political agenda (Hawe *et al.* 1995). But because much of our economy is health-based and the discourse of health is so powerful, different groups and institutions have interests in how health and public health are conceptualized.

The face of public health has changed over time depending on the dominant disease patterns and the status of scientific advances and technological know-how to combat these. From the seventeenth to the nineteenth centuries, public health was preoccupied with eliminating diseases such as the plague, cholera and smallpox, which posed a threat to a large number of people. With industrialization and rapid urbanization in the nineteenth century, public health gained a broader vision, dealing with all aspects of environmental sanitation, including living conditions, mainly with the aim of securing a functioning working population (Lewis 1986). The bacteriological revolution and further scientific advances in the late nineteenth and early twentieth centuries shifted attention away from the social and structural causes of ill health towards personal hygiene and an increased interest in the 'healthy body' (Lewis 1986). Subsequently, three post-war eras led to the development of a health promotion policy in the USA: 'the era of resource development', which produced a disease-focused medical infrastructure; 'the era of redistribution', which introduced laws to give consumers medical purchasing power and used health education to increase health service utilization; and 'the cost containment era', which aimed to control costs by decreasing the need for medical care and used health education to target appropriate use of health services and to advocate self-care (Green and Kreuter 1991). The term 'health promotion' emerged in US health policy in 1975, it is said, as a last minute substitute for the term health education, merely to avoid having the bills referred to the education committees where they would have died for lack of interest or priority (Green and Kreuter 1991). The publication of the 'Lalonde Report' (Lalonde 1974) in Canada and the 'Healthy People Report' (US Surgeon General 1979) in the USA institutionalized a vision that disease was strongly, although not exclusively, associated with controllable risk factors rooted in individual behaviour. The locus for change that might improve the public health clearly shifted away from social factors, such as housing, employment and income, to individual psychological factors, such as coping, social support and healthy lifestyle (Research Unit in Health and Behavioural Change 1995). Though public health strategies at the levels of institutional change, legislation and policy were included, they proved difficult to implement, especially in an era of fiscal conservatism (Minkler 1989). As citizen participation and self-care had taken the shape of a significant social movement, and represented a welcome relief for programme budgets, it was a short step for public health to shift its emphasis from institution building and centrally planned programmes to self-reliance, person-centred initiatives and individual participation in health (Green and Kreuter 1991). An additional advantage of stressing the individual approach was the voluntary nature of interventions that ensued and the protection of the right to choose one's lifestyle, as opposed to the coercive tendency of state interventions trying to assert the interests, rights and obligations of the community against the individual (Yeo 1993).

The notion of health promotion in Europe had its origins in 1980 when the World Health Organization (WHO) Regional Office recognized that health education in isolation from other measures would not necessarily result in radical changes in health, and introduced a range of non-educational approaches which were designated 'health promotion' (Parish 1996). These centred on health as 'a complete state of physical, mental and social well-being and not merely the absence of disease', and focused on the social, political and economic determinants of health not amenable to improvement by medical care (Robertson and Minkler 1994). As such, health promotion provides an alternative to the medicalized notion of health, and aims to go beyond individual lifestyle strategies. Though it is often thought of as a 'new' concept, a development of the 'new public health' of the 1970s and 1980s, some authors argue that it is merely a 'renaissance' of a broad and encompassing concept of public health (Green and Kreuter 1991).

Similar trends in public health, from environmental engineering to health education, occurred in the UK (Bunton and MacDonald 1992). The first

Public Health Act emerged in 1848 as a direct result of the recognition that there is a relationship between poverty and ill health, linked to bad sanitation at home and at work. The second Public Health Act in 1872 created local medical officers of health, who initially had a broad remit to include sanitation and housing, but gradually drifted towards the biomedical aspects and lifestyle determinants of illness and disease. Health education in the UK started with the establishment of the Central Council for Health Education in 1927, for which the Society of Medical Officers of Health had lobbied. The principle functions of the Council were 'to promote and encourage education . . . in the science and art of healthy living', and 'to coordinate the work of all statutory bodies in carrying out their powers and duties under the Public Health Acts . . . relating to the promotion . . . of Public Health' (Bunton and MacDonald 1992: 10). While the Council took the first function to heart, mainly concentrating on lifestyle, it neglected the second, mainly ignoring structural approaches. Upon its foundation in 1948, the National Health Service (NHS) contributed about 50 per cent of its budget to local authority health education work (Sutherland 1987). After the 1974 NHS reorganization, however, health education became the responsibility of health authorities and was 'officially' separated from environmental health, which remained the responsibility of the local authorities. This separation further enhanced the medical dominance of health education. Though the Health Education Council in 1981 preferred to use the term 'health promotion' rather than 'health education', recognition of the fact that determinants of health were broader than just lifestyle (Health Education Council 1983) had little impact on policy. The emphasis on individuals rather than structures was continued with the publication of the *Health of the Nation* document by the Department of Health in the early nineties (Thomas 1993). Despite the medicalization of 'health promotion', particularly as it was practised by health professionals as an adjunct to their clinical care, health promotion attracted new specialists and voluntary sector workers who shared anti-authoritarian attitudes, were sympathetic to social science critiques of health promotion and favoured community empowerment approaches (Kelly and Charlton 1992). It is only recently that the UK government has refocused its attention to better health on a concerted action between national and local players, as well as the general public.

What principles underpin health promotion?

A large body of evidence has demonstrated the relationship between socio-economic status and disease (Black *et al.* 1980; Whitehead 1992; Feinstein 1993; Kreiger *et al.* 1993; Davey Smith *et al.* 1994; Acheson 1998), but the gap between the health status of rich and poor is becoming wider still.

Logically, this means that giving special consideration to disadvantaged population groups and changing their social and material context is not only an ethical imperative, but also a promising route to better public health. According to Yeo (1993), health promotion ethics essentially needs to address two main issues: 'distributive justice' and 'intervention ethics'. Distributive justice is aimed at clarifying principles and values for allocating resources to health, one of which is reducing inequity in health status within and across populations. Intervention ethics deals with assessing various health promotion interventions for their impact on cherished values such as privacy, freedom, responsibility and the common good (Yeo 1993). Intervention ethics could also, and perhaps foremost, address the fundamental admonition of 'first do no harm'.

The Ottawa Charter for Health Promotion (1986), which emerged out of the first International Conference on Health Promotion, acknowledged that the basic prerequisites for any improvement in health are peace, shelter, education, food, income, a stable ecosystem, sustainable resources, social justice and equity, but how these are to be obtained is less obvious. Two decades later, the two million children that still die each year from diseases for which there are effective vaccines are testament to the lack of political will and commitment from individual governments as well as the international community to reducing these tolls (Nakajima 1998). Most of these deaths occur in developing countries, few of which have reaped the public health or other benefits of technological advances. Some argue that epidemiology has dominated and is still pivotal to public health teaching and practice, while the social sciences, which stress a broader view including social conscience, are largely ignored (Research Unit in Health and Behavioural Change 1995). Greater attention to the social sciences is, however, shown in health promotion today.

The centrepiece of the health promotion paradigm is the concept of empowerment – enabling people to increase control over and to improve their own health. Empowerment claims to attribute responsibility to people not for the existence of the problem, but for finding a solution to it. The goal is then 'full and organised community participation and ultimate self-reliance' (Yeo 1993: 233). Health promotion perceives the community as a setting or social system that has the potential to act as a resource to promote health from the bottom up (Macdonald and Davies 1998). The role of the health promotion professional is only to facilitate the strengthening or building of such communities. Some go as far as claiming that 'If the activity under consideration is not enabling and empowering then it is not health promotion' (Macdonald and Davies 1998). The vehicles for operationalizing this approach are based on settings where people live and work, such as Healthy Cities and Health Promoting Schools (Macdonald and Davies 1998). However, the extent to which its key strategies of empowerment and community participation have improved people's lives or their health remains virtually undocumented. In addition, little or no guidance is provided on how to deal with potential conflicts over perceived needs and resources between different communities and stakeholders, or between the agenda of the community and the larger agenda of equity and social justice (Robertson and Minkler 1994).

Health promotion, in essence, seeks to effect changes in the health behaviour of individuals. Health promotion practitioners are often eclectic in practice, using varied conceptual models for understanding and modifying behaviour, research methodologies and differing philosophical frameworks for contextualizing risk and protective behaviours associated with health promotion and disease prevention (DiClemente and Raczynski 1999). A wide range of theories and models have been developed to explain the factors that determine behaviour and the mechanisms by which they do so, such as the health belief model (Rosenstock 1974), the theory of reasoned action (Ajzen and Fishbein 1980), social-cognitive theory (Bandura 1986), the transtheoretical model of change (Prochaska and DiClemente 1986), the persuasion communication model (McGuire 1985), attribution theory (Weiner 1986), social network and social support theories (Gottlieb 1985) and the diffusion of innovations theory (Rogers 1995). This wide-ranging literature has led to some confusion about how theory can be used to guide the development, implementation and evaluation of health promotion interventions. Indeed, some argue that

> attempts to change health-related behaviours by health educators and others have largely failed because of undue reliance on the literature of social psychology and the application of models of behavioural change which owe more to the cooperation of American college students than they do to an understanding of the context and complexity of the phenomenon itself.
>
> (Research Unit in Health and Behavioural Change 1995: 67)

Although psychological theories have contributed to our understanding of how to motivate and maintain behaviour change, there is a need for health promotion programmes to incorporate more structural alterations (Macdonald and Davies 1998). A particularly useful contribution to the theoretical underpinning of health education and health promotion practice was presented by Bartholomew and colleagues (2001), who gave an overview of behaviour-oriented theories, mostly from behavioural sciences, environment-oriented theories and the socio-political sciences, mapped on to 'ecological' levels. The social ecological paradigm focuses on the interrelationships between individuals, with their biological, psychological and behavioural characteristics, and the physical, social and cultural aspects that exist across the individual's life domains and social settings. 'The picture that emerges is a complex Web of causation as well as a rich context for intervention; looking for the most effective leverage points within this Web, across levels, reduces the complexity and is necessary for the development of effective multi-level interventions' (Bartholomew *et al.* 2001: 5).

An intervention method, then, is a defined process by which theory postulates how change may occur in the behaviour of an individual, a small group, or a social structure; and the translation of selected intervention methods into action is completed through the development of strategies, i.e. ways of organizing and operationalizing the methods (Bartholomew *et al.* 2001). For example, to increase fruit and vegetable consumption by children in the school canteen, methods of persuasion and modelling may be used to influence the purchasing practices of the food service manager. Strategies may include testimonials by food service personnel from other schools who already have incorporated healthier buying practices (Bartholomew *et al.* 2001). While health interventions can occur at many different levels (e.g. the individual, the family, the neighbourhood, the worksite, the organization, the community, the city), health interventions essentially have two basic targets: factors within the control of the individual, and factors outside the individual's control (Cohen *et al.* 2000). Interventions targeting the latter are underutilized approaches for improving the nation's health. However, some have claimed that 'the individualistic approach will persist . . . because however misguided, [it] is less costly politically as well as for programme budgets, and for economies – at least in the short term' (Yeo 1993: 399).

Challenges from medicine

Three major challenges face health promotion in the UK: competition from medicine for funds; the appeal and convenience of individualistic approaches for their apparent simplicity and low cost; and the medical dominance of NHS policy and practice. The dominant vision among health promoters today is that too much emphasis has been placed on the health care system – relabelled by some a 'sickness care' system – and that priorities need to be re-examined. Taking the field of HIV/AIDS as an example, Hunter and Chen (1992: 399) pointed out back in 1988:

> It has become almost banal to assert that in the absence of an effective vaccine or treatment, education is the only weapon against the AIDS epidemic. Yet most funding worldwide still goes to clinical or laboratory research . . . Possible causes include lack of communication between the competing scientific cultures of the biomedical and social sciences, the influence in AIDS funding decisions of representatives of developed countries trained to look for technological solutions, and the frequent dominance of medically trained scientists with the same technological orientation in national AIDS committees in all countries.

More than ten years on, nothing much has changed in the balance between medicine and health promotion, and we are still waiting, unfortunately, for a technological solution to HIV/AIDS. As mentioned above, the NHS in the UK contributed about 50 per cent of its budget to local authority health education work in 1948 (Sutherland 1987). In 1996, on the other hand, spending on health promotion represented less than 1 per cent of the NHS annual budget, and less than the expenditure in staff cars and travelling and subsistence in 1995–6 (Speller *et al.* 1997).

Health promotion clearly needs to assert itself, but is further challenged by the medical dominance of policy and practice. Much health promotion practice is carried out by clinicians such as doctors, nurses, dentists and pharmacists, and health promotion policy falls within the management of consultants of public health medicine. These groups have been strongly influenced by the emergence of evidence-based practice as one of the dominant themes within the NHS in the UK.

The provision of health care is about making decisions, which often involves choosing between a number of alternative actions. In health promotion, there is a wide choice of interventions involving a range of professionals, practitioners and policy makers in different settings – from health care workers targeting individual behaviour to politicians making policies on employment, housing conditions, transport and so on, that potentially contribute to improving health, preventing disease and reducing social inequalities. In making a decision on where to allocate resources, we can draw on a wide variety of information, such as professional or personal experience, client preferences, external rules and constraints, and scientific evidence. Appleby and colleagues (1995: 5) state that 'evidence-based health care in essence involves a shift in the culture of health care provision, away from basing decisions on opinion, past practice and precedent, and towards making more use of science, research and evidence to guide decision-making.' Definitions of evidence-based practice vary, but they all have in common the drive to make informed decisions based, at least in part, on the best available evidence, i.e. sound evidence from rigorous research where available. No advocates of evidence-based health care would argue that evidence dictates what should be done in any particular circumstance, but instead they stress that research findings should always be considered together with the preferences of clients and professional judgement. Even in cases for which evidence is difficult to find or poor in quality, the decision-maker must search for it, appraise and present it, even if the decision taken may ultimately be dominated by values and resources (Gray 1997).

The problem of access to research evidence and skills for critically appraising it is a recurrent one, and fundamental to evidence-based policy and practice.

Anyone with the responsibility to help individuals and communities change health risk behaviour, initiate health-promoting behaviour, change environmental factors, or manage illness must design or adapt existing effective interventions and develop plans to implement them. Yet there remains some confusion about how planners can integrate the wealth of information, theories, ideas, and models to develop interventions that are logical and appropriate in their foundations and are practical and acceptable in their administration. Seldom do health educators write in depth about the process of intervention development, and complicated interventions are often reduced to several sentences in evaluation articles.

(Bartholomew *et al.* 2001: 8)

Conducting, maintaining and disseminating systematic reviews of the effects of health care, including health promotion, is a logical step in the progress towards evidence-based health care. Systematic reviews are a short-cut to accessing and integrating the findings across individual studies. They differ from 'traditional' literature reviews in their methods, which consistently aim to limit potential bias and other errors. These methods are explicitly reported so that others can assess the integrity of the review process and, hence, the validity of the review. The very task of conducting systematic reviews, and thus increasing access to the best available evidence, has become the focus of a rapidly growing international group of individuals from a wide variety of backgrounds (including clinicians, sociologists, methodologists and consumers) who have formed the Cochrane Collaboration. The Cochrane Collaboration aims to help people to make well informed decisions about health care by preparing, maintaining and promoting the accessibility of systematic reviews of the effects of health care interventions. So far, more than 900 systematic reviews on the effects of a variety of health care interventions have been completed and over 800 are in progress. These reviews, together with other resources, are widely disseminated as *The Cochrane Library* on CD-ROM or on-line (http://update.cochrane.co.uk). The Cochrane Field of Health Promotion and Public Health aims to facilitate the full integration of health promotion in evidence-based health care. Several systematic reviews of the effectiveness of health promotion interventions have been compiled (see Chapter 3). However, they have not always been received well, especially by health promotion practitioners (see also Chapter 11). This has been mainly due to criticism of the type of evidence incorporated in those reviews: primarily randomized controlled trials (RCTs).

Challenges to trials

Within the UK, as in many other parts of Europe, and in the USA, health promotion had to cope with a greater emphasis on monitoring and evaluation, in addition to other pressures. The view that evidence-based health service agendas are associated with new approaches to rationing is widespread (House 1993). In addition, there is concern about an over-concentration on outcome measures and quantitative data, which are seen by many as an outmoded and inappropriate way to measure the effectiveness of health promotion programmes (Macdonald and Davies 1998). Objective measures of health are often viewed as precluding one of the principles of health promotion: that communities should be involved in developing their own notions of positive health (Hancock 1993). Overall, there appears to be a tension between the focus of health promotion on subjective health and more standard definitions of preventing disease and illness, including economic considerations. Attempts to compare the cost-effectiveness of different interventions have been seen as having limited practical value because of the inevitable lack of comparability of outcomes between different projects (Burrows *et al.* 1995). Many evaluation techniques have been accused of being based on an unrealistic idea of what health promotion could or even should achieve (Macdonald and Davies 1998).

Towner and colleagues (1993) have specifically cautioned against RCTs being seen as the 'gold standard' in evaluating health promotion, since this may draw attention towards certain types of approaches, especially those targeting individual behaviour, which are not necessarily more effective but can be more easily evaluated with RCT designs. In addition, health promotion specialists have argued that it is often impossible to demonstrate causal links owing to the complex interplay of variables; and that there are inevitable time lags related to health status outcomes, often inter-generational. Essentially what critics are arguing is that

> health promotion programmes and interventions need to be assessed in relation to the social and structural influences that determine health. They therefore need to adopt an approach to evaluation that implicitly acknowledges the need for outcome data but explicitly concentrates on process or illuminative data that helps us understand the nature of that relationship.
>
> (Macdonald and Davies 1998: 6)

There is an additional concern that, while health promotion aims to empower and should be participative, research is often developed in a non-participative manner. Alternative approaches to research that are action-oriented and community-controlled have been proposed (Hancock 1993). At first sight these are at odds with the application of the RCT design, with its standardized health outcome measures and the lack of appropriate emphasis on the practicalities of mounting health interventions. However, there are now several good examples of community-based RCTs, and other experimental designs, that have incorporated the needs of the targeted community, have invited the community to play an active role in the development and delivery of appropriate interventions and have included qualitative methods which can offer critical and illuminating evidence of what happens during a programme. Several chapters in this book discuss these issues in more detail.

Evidence-based health care has developed in parallel with the growth of consumer involvement in health and 'patient power', with raised expectations for high-quality services and a justification of decisions made by health care providers (CASP 1999). This empowerment of individuals and communities requires professionals to be frank about the effectiveness of a particular intervention, and to provide comprehensive information in an appropriate way to those targeted by the intervention in order to enable them to share in the decision-making. Although clinicians place the patient at the centre of evidence-based health care, there is a tendency for them to project their own understanding of patient priorities rather than allowing patients to set the agenda. As patients' opportunities for making their own choices increase, evidence-based medicine is challenged in much the same way as it has itself challenged health promotion. In fact, health promotion can draw on its longstanding experience with action research and community participation methods to make an important contribution to evidence-based health care. Here is an excellent opportunity for health promotion to take a leading role, rather than trailing behind medicine, in one of the central issues of evidence-based decision-making, one to which medicine has only recently opened itself up and has few lessons to offer: how to integrate the client perspective and methodological pluralism (combining qualitative and quantitative methods) in issues of effectiveness. Isn't the aim to take the best of what we know and put it to use in a concerted effort to make a real difference in people's lives? As Bartholomew and colleagues (2001: 7) put it, 'The emphasis in health promotion is on participation, with a commitment to bringing both a community and a multi-disciplinary professional perspective to bear on a problem and create the most intelligent, productive consensus possible on the planning and conduct of health promotion activities.'

Conclusions

The key messages of this chapter are:

- Health promotion goes beyond a focus on individual lifestyles, to take into account the broader determinants of health. It goes beyond the perspectives of professionals, to include the active participation of communities.
- Evidence-informed policy and practice makes decisions based on the best available research evidence, moderated by client circumstances and drawing on professionals' expertise, skills and judgement.

This book is rooted in the fundamental principles of both health promotion and evidence-informed policy and practice and offers suggestions for reconciling apparent conflicts between the two. Health promotion has a unique opportunity to contribute to evidence-based methods, leading the way in how the client perspective and a methodological pluralism can be integrated in issues of effectiveness.

References

Acheson, D. (1998) *Independent Inquiry into Inequalities in Health Report*. London: The Stationery Office.

Aggleton, P. (1997) Health education. *AIDS Care*, 9, 35–9.

Appleby, J., Walshe, K. and Ham, C. (1995) *Acting on the Evidence: a Review of Clinical Effectiveness: Sources of Information, Dissemination and Implementation*. Birmingham: National Association of Health Authorities and Trusts, Health Services Management Centre, University of Birmingham.

Ajzen, I. and Fishbein, M. (1980) *Understanding Attitudes and Predicting Social Behavior*. Englewood Cliffs, NJ: Prentice Hall.

Bandura, A. (1986) *Social Foundations of Thought and Action. A Social Cognitive Theory*. Englewood Cliffs, NJ: Prentice Hall.

Bartholomew, L., Parcel, G., Kok, G. and Gottlieb, N. (2001) *Intervention Mapping. Designing Theory- and Evidence-based Health Promotion*. Mountain View, CA: Mayfield Publishing Company.

Black, D., Morris, J., Smith, C. and Townsend, P. (1980) *The Black Report*. London: Penguin Books.

Bunton, R. and Macdonald, G. (1992) *Health Promotion. Disciplines and Diversity*. London: Routledge.

Burrows, R., Bunton, R., Muncer, S. and Gillen, K. (1995) The efficacy of health promotion: health economics and late modernism. *Health Education Research*, 10(2), 241–9.

CASP (1999) Evidence-based health care. An open learning resource for health care practitioners. Critical Appraisal Skills Programme and Health Care Libraries Unit. NHS Executive Anglia and Oxford.

Cohen, D., Scribner, R. and Farley, T. (2000) A structural model of health behavior: a pragmatic approach to explain and influence health behaviors at the population level. *Preventive Medicine*, 30, 146–54.

Davey Smith, G., Blane, D. and Bartley, M. (1994) Explanations for socio-economic differentials in mortality. Evidence from Britain and elsewhere. *European Journal of Public Health*, 4(2), 131–44.

Devers, K. (1999) How will we know 'good' qualitative research when we see it? Beginning the dialogue in health services research. *Health Services Research*, 34(5), 1153–88.

DiClemente, R. and Raczynski, J. (1999) The importance of health promotion and disease prevention. In J. Raczynski and R. DiClemente (eds) *Handbook of Health Promotion and Disease Prevention*. New York: Plenum Publishers.

Feinstein, S. (1993) The relationship between socio-economic status and health: a review of the literature. *Milbank Quarterly*, 71(2), 279–322.

Gottlieb, N. (1985) Social networks and social support: an overview of research, practice, and policy implementations. *Health Education Quarterly*, 12(1), 5–22.

Gray, J. (1997) *Evidence-based Healthcare. How to Make Health Policy and Management Decisions*. London: Churchill Livingstone.

Green, L. and Kreuter, M. (1991) *Health Promotion Planning: An Educational and Environmental Approach*. Mountain View, CA: Mayfield Publishing Company.

Hancock, T. (1993) The Healthy City: from concept to application. In J. Davies and M. Kelly (eds) *Healthy Cities: Research and Practice*. London: Routledge.

Hawe, P., Degeling, D. and Hall, J. (1995) *Evaluating Health Promotion: A Health Worker's Guide*. Sydney: MacLennan and Petty.

Health Education Council (1983) *Healthy Living. Towards a National Strategy for Health Education and Health Promotion*. London: Health Education Council.

House, E. (1993) *Professional Evaluation: Social Impact and Political Consequences*. London: Sage.

Hunter, D. and Chen, L. (1992) The impact of AIDS, and AIDS education, in the context of health problems in the developing world. In J. Sepulveda, H. Fineberg and J. Manns (eds) *AIDS – Prevention through Education: A World View*. New York: Oxford University Press.

Kelly, M. and Charlton, B. (1992) Health promotion: time for a new philosophy? *British Journal of General Practice*, June, 223–4.

Kirby, D., Short, L., Collins, J. *et al.* (1994) School-based programs to reduce sexual risk behaviors: a review of effectiveness. *Public Health Reports*, 3, 339–61.

Kitson, A., Ahmed, L., Harvey, G., Seers, K. and Thompson, D. (1996) From research to practice: one organisational model for promoting research based practice. *Journal of Advanced Nursing*, 23, 430–40.

Kreiger, N., Rowley, D. and Herman, A. (1993) Racism, sexism, and social class: implications for studies of health, disease, and well-being. *American Journal of Public Health*, 83(1), 82–122.

Lalonde, M. (1974) *A New Perspective on the Health of Canadians*. Ottawa: Government of Canada.

Lewis, J. (1986) *What Price Community Medicine? The Philosophy, Practice and Politics of Public Health since 1919*. Brighton: Harvester.

Macdonald, G. and Davies, J. (1998) Reflection and vision. Proving and improving the promotion of health. In J. Davies and G. Macdonald (eds) *Quality, Evidence and Effectiveness in Health Promotion. Striving for Certainties*. London: Routledge.

McGuire, W. (1985) Attitudes and attitude changes. In G. Lindzey and E. Aronson (eds) *The Handbook of Social Psychology. Volume 2, Special Fields and Applications*. New York: Knopf.

Minkler, M. (1989) Health education, health promotion and the open society: an historical perspective. *Health Education Quarterly*, 16(1), 17–30.

Nakajima, H. (1998) Message from the Director General. In *The World Health Report 1998. Life in the 21st Century: A Vision for All*. Geneva: World Health Organization.

Oakley, A. (1998) Personal views: living in two worlds. *British Medical Journal*, 316, 482–3.

Oakley, A. (2000) *Experiments in Knowing. Gender and Methodology in the Social Sciences*. Cambridge: Polity Press.

Oakley, A., Fullerton, D., Holland, J. *et al.* (1995) Sexual health education interventions for young people: a methodological review. *British Medical Journal*, 310, 158–62.

Ottawa Charter for Health Promotion (1986) *Health Promotion*, 1(4), i–v.

Parish, R. (1996) Health promotion. Rhetoric and reality. In R. Bunton, S. Nettleton and R. Burrows (eds) *The Sociology of Health Promotion. Critical Analyses of Consumption, Lifestyle and Risk.* London: Routledge.

Peersman, G., Oakley, A., Oliver, S. and Thomas, J. (1996) *Review of Effectiveness of Sexual Health Promotion Interventions for Young People.* London: EPI-Centre, Social Science Research Unit.

Prochaska, J. and DiClemente, C. (1986) Toward a comprehensive model of change, in W. Miller and N. Heather (eds) *Treating Addictive Behaviors: Processes of Change.* New York: Plenum Press.

Research Unit in Health and Behavioural Change, University of Edinburgh (1995) *Changing the Public Health.* Chichester: John Wiley & Sons.

Robertson, A. and Minkler, M. (1994) New health promotion movement: a critical examination. *Health Education Quarterly*, 21(3), 295–312.

Rogers, E. (1995) *Diffusion of innovations.* New York: Free Press.

Rosenstock, I. (1974) Historical origins of the health belief model. *Health Education Monographs*, 2, 328–35.

Sackett, D., Scott Richardson, W., Rosenberg, W. and Haynes, B. (1997) *Evidence-based Medicine. How to Practise and Teach EBM.* London: Churchill Livingstone.

Speller, V., Learmonth, A. and Harrison, D. (1997) The search for evidence of effective health promotion. *British Medical Journal*, 315, 361–3.

Sutherland, I. (1987) *Health Education: Half a Policy. The Rise and Fall of the Health Education Council.* Cambridge: National Extension College.

Thomas, C. (1993) Public health strategies in Sheffield and England: a comparison of conceptual foundations. *Health Promotion International*, 8(4), 299–307.

Towner, E., Dowswell, T. and Jarvis, S. (1993) *Reducing Childhood Accidents. The Effectiveness of Health Promotion Interventions: A Literature Review.* London: Health Education Authority.

US Surgeon General (1979) *Healthy People: The Surgeon General's Report on Health Promotion and Disease Prevention.* Washington, DC: Department of Health and Human Services.

Weiner, B. (1986) *An Attributional Theory of Motivation and Emotion.* New York: Springer.

Whitehead, M. (1992) *The Health Divide.* London: Penguin Books.

WHO (1998) *The World Health Report 1998. Life in the 21st Century: A Vision for All.* Geneva: World Health Organization.

Wight, D. (1997) School-based sex education. *AIDS Care*, 9, 35–9.

Yeo, M. (1993) Toward an ethic of empowerment for health promotion. *Health Promotion International*, 8(3), 225–35.

Ziglio, E. (1996) How to move towards evidence-based health promotion interventions. Paper presented at the Third European Conference on Effectiveness, Turin, 12–14 September.

▶ **2**

▷ Evaluating health promotion: methodological diversity

▷ **Ann Oakley**

The following story about the origins of evaluation is quoted from Michael Patton's *Creative Evaluation*:

> In the beginning God created the heaven and the earth . . .
> And God saw everything He made. 'Behold,' God said, 'it is very good'.
> And the evening and the morning were the sixth day.
> And on the seventh day God rested from all his work.
> His archangel came then unto Him asking:
> 'God, how do you know what you have created is "very good"? What are your criteria?
> On what data do you base your judgement? Aren't you a little close to the situation to make a fair and unbiased evaluation?'
> God thought about these questions all that day and His rest was greatly disturbed.
> On the eighth day God said, 'Lucifer, go to hell.'
> Thus was evaluation born in a blaze of glory.
>
> (Peberdy 1997a: 269)

This story has several significant features. First, and as Peberdy (1997a: 270) points out, the project manager and the evaluator are different actors who are coming at the issue from different viewpoints. While the project manager (God) is convinced of the value of his intervention, the evaluator (the archangel) asks awkward questions about the basis of this conviction. Second, after some reflection, the project manager decides to go on believing what he wants to, without bothering about the evaluator's questions. Third, this disjunction between perspectives does not impede the birth of a whole new industry – that of evaluation.

This chapter looks at the real origins of evaluation as an industry, examines some of the different arguments about how it might be applied to health promotion and discusses some examples of different evaluation strategies, together with their implications for health promotion's knowledge-base.

Evaluating interventions

Attempts to improve people's health encompass prevention, treatment and rehabilitation. They may target individuals or communities, be aimed at health knowledge, attitudes, values or behaviours, and consist of either clinical or social interventions. Health promotion is an example of a social intervention. It thus belongs to a much wider category of actions performed by a range of professionals and others which are designed to bring about a variety of different kinds of change in people's lives. When some people do something to other people, a number of questions are typically prompted. What are they doing it *for*? *How* are they doing it, to *whom* and *why*? What do the *recipients* think of it? Does it *work*? Does it do any *harm*? How much does it *cost*? Last but not least, how do we *know*?

All these questions have historically been asked of both clinical and social interventions. However, the implementation, impact and history of clinical interventions have received considerably more attention than those of social interventions. The central challenge in evaluating clinical interventions, that of establishing effectiveness, dates from at least the mid-sixteenth century, although this did not really take root as a major professional concern until the 1940s (Oakley 2000; see also www.rcpe.ac.uk for continuously updated references to early examples). More recently, the international Cochrane Collaboration has developed procedures for collecting and synthesizing evidence which make it possible for health care workers to base their practice on an open, systematic and quality-assured knowledge base (Chalmers *et al.* 1997). The accessibility of the resulting knowledge is potentially a major influence on the traditional hierarchical relationship between users and providers of health care, pushing it in a more democratic direction (Goodare and Lockwood 1999; Oliver 1999). All professionals have a tendency to claim exclusive ownership of relevant knowledge, so when this knowledge is in the public domain and collected according to transparent principles, professionals find it harder simply to do what they think is best, without also taking into account their clients' perspectives.

The drive towards assembling reliable evidence in medicine has been part of a much broader cultural move towards a 'scientific' understanding of human social relations. Central to this endeavour has been the desire to grasp relationships between cause and effect. This in turn has meant developing procedures which help to rule out the operations of chance (Hacking 1990).

It was this same impetus which gave birth in the nineteenth and early twentieth centuries to a quantitative social science. Social science took as one of its tasks the challenge of appraising the efforts of those who sought to improve human life. To this end a variety of methods were used: large-scale surveys, interviews and observational work, case studies and experimental designs. 'Scientific' or 'laboratory' sociology was an established preoccupation by the early 1900s. Such fields as education, criminology, health promotion and social welfare came to be marked by a significant attention to questions about effectiveness, which yielded a focus on measurement and experimentation (McCall 1923; Greenwood 1945; Chapin 1947). In the USA this tradition was later extended to a number of large-scale government-funded social experiments, where such interventions as income maintenance, housing allowances, re-employment and training schemes, free or subsidized health care and pre-school education were tested for their capacity to improve welfare, health, educational and employment outcomes for mainly socially disadvantaged populations (Boruch and Riecken 1975; Ferber and Hirsch 1982; Miller and Lewis 1987; Boruch 1997; see also Oakley 2000).

Significantly, the US government mandated that a condition of such spending was that a proportion should be spent on well designed evaluations of programme effectiveness and acceptability. The context that gave rise to this decision was an interesting example of the belief that accessible, quality-assured evidence can be a major force for more equal social relations. Worried that federal money provided for disadvantaged children would be spent by educators without any significant impact on outcome, Senator Robert Kennedy attached an evaluation clause to the Elementary and Secondary Education Act of 1965. This led to evaluation of the initiative, and forced schools to provide test scores to parents, so that parents could monitor school performance (McLaughlin 1975).

The American experience of social experimentation provides many unique examples of the difficult relationship between research and policy (Nathan 1988). Policy is rarely informed by research findings in any linear way, even when the policy makers commissioned the research in the first place. The American experience also shows that the so-called methods of the natural sciences are perfectly feasible in social settings. In applying these approaches to social interventions, evaluators pioneered some key events in the history of evaluation methodology in general. These include work on the validity of different experimental designs (Campbell and Stanley 1963), and appropriate procedures for meta-analysis, or synthesizing the results of different evaluations in combined estimates of the extent to which interventions may or may not have been effective (Hunt 1997). The early development of this procedure – an important element in health care research reviews – came about as a response to conflicting findings about the impact of the Head Start programme for disadvantaged children in the USA (Light and Smith 1971). It was later developed to settle a dispute about the benefits of psychotherapy (Glass *et al.* 1981). What is significant about these developments is that they arose in the social, not the medical, domain.

Despite this history, anyone who works in health promotion today will be aware that the use of experimental designs to evaluate social interventions is a highly contested area.

Paradigm wars

The primary contest is often framed as between those who espouse 'medical' and those who advocate 'social' models of research and evaluation (see, for example, Green and Kreuter 1991; Bunton and Macdonald 1992; Downie *et al.* 1996; Peberdy 1997a; Oakley 1999, 2000 for discussions). Alan Beattie (1997: 234) puts it like this:

> For much of the past fifteen years, different approaches to evaluation have been polarised into two warring camps. On the one hand there have been the various traditions of quantitative evaluation – drawing either on scientific research in experimental or quasi-experimental modes, or on managerial audits using statistical or other numerical ways of 'figuring out performance' in terms of economy, efficiency and effectiveness. On the other hand there emerged – largely outside the worlds of medical research and management sciences and unknown to them – a range of alternative 'qualitative' strategies of evaluation which focused on the portrayal of people, places and processes through ethnographic and other kinds of description.

The dispute about method has yielded some vehement positioning, notably in relation to 'positivism', which appears most often as a term of abuse (see, for example, Stevenson and Burke 1991; Davies and Macdonald 1998). 'Evidence-based everything' (Carr-Hill 1995) or 'the holy grail' of evidence-based medicine (Williams and Popay 1997) come in for special attack. Randomized controlled trials (RCTs), under a variety of nomenclatures, including 'random controlled' and 'randomized control' trial, are frequently cited as a disfavoured form of inquiry. Davies and Macdonald (1998: 209) describe the objection to the RCT in the following terms: 'Its underlying ideology is expert driven, authoritarian and disempowering; seeking evidence through narrow clinically based methods and short-term quantitative outcome measures.' A central objection is that the values underlying RCTs are at odds with those of health promotion as a form of social action based on principles of community participation and empowerment. Thus, a description of the processes involved in developing, implementing and appraising health promotion interventions, 'action' research or 'illuminative' evaluation focuses on internal day-to-day structures in particular settings may be held up as a more appropriate way of answering the questions that need to be asked about their impact (Scott 1992; Tones 1997; de Ven and Aggleton 1999).

The paradigm war features prominently in the European methods literature from the 1960s (Bryman 1988). It was preceded by something very similar in the 1930s in the USA, where the competition between Chicago and Columbia schools of social science produced some very modern-sounding statements about the denial of subjective experience and rigid adherence to measurement for its own sake implied in natural science methods (though the favoured term of abuse then was 'behaviourism', not 'positivism': Bain 1931; Lundberg 1933).

The argument about methods for evaluating interventions is part of a broader dissension between 'quantitative' and 'qualitative' ways of knowing (Bulmer 1984; Silverman 1985; Bryman 1988). It can be hard to tell what the essential disagreement is, though ideology, philosophy, values, beliefs, principles and practice have all been implicated. An important way of 'reading' the methods war is to ask oneself what the terms being bandied about *really* mean. For example, when people talk critically about 'empiricist' or 'positivist' methods, condemn the 'biomedical model' or reject a 'hierarchy of evidence', what substantive points are they making about evaluation methodology, and to what extent might these be borne out or not by the way evaluations have in practice been done?

What is evaluation?

Given such disagreement, it is clearly important to take a hard look at the meaning of evaluation, and to consider how it can be applied to best effect in the domain of health promotion.

The most economical way of defining evaluation is as 'the process that will enable us to learn from experience' (Turner *et al.* 1989: 316). Different approaches are tried: for example, to prevent young people taking up smoking; to encourage gay men to engage in safer-sex behaviours; to promote the principle of community involvement in the care of the environment; to reducing accidents among children; or to persuading people to eat more healthy food. But these endeavours cannot yield clear lessons unless there has been some attempt at cumulative analytical description. Evaluation can thus also be seen as a set of procedures which judge 'the worth of an activity' (Peberdy 1997b: 73). It is something we all do in everyday life, and it has two essential components: setting standards against which the doing of something can be judged; and deciding whether or not the activity in question meets those standards. Most evaluation criteria (standards) fall under five headings: *effectiveness*, the extent to which stated goals are met; *appropriateness*, the relationship to need; *acceptability*, to the recipients; *equity*, whether there is equal provision for those with the same needs; and *efficiency*, a criterion which involves some calculation of relative costs and benefits (Philips *et al.* 1994).

The term 'evaluation' covers studies which aim to describe both *processes* and *outcomes*; that is, to answer questions about why something happens as well as those about whether it works or not (Coyle *et al.* 1991). Evaluation research is a subset of research in general. This means that there are other important research questions which are not directly related to implementation or effectiveness, the dominant concerns of evaluation. For example, researchers may want to know how people prioritize different health promotion topics; they may want to study the interrelationships between the way people live and the extent to which their behaviours are health-promoting; they may be interested in collecting data in order to develop theories, models or conceptual understandings. While each of these can be part of an evaluation study (see below for some examples), they also form standalone enquiries.

Evaluation in practice

One way to look at the range of methods used to evaluate health promotion is through a systematic study of the literature in a particular area. Table 2.1 shows the results of such a mapping exercise carried out in 1996 for young people and six specific health promotion topics. Electronic databases were searched for relevant literature published between 1983 and 1995, and the titles and abstracts thus obtained were then classified by topic area and research design. In Table 2.1 *descriptive studies* include needs assessment, cross-sectional surveys, case–control studies, cohort studies and reviews; *outcome evaluations* means evaluations designed to establish whether an intervention changed health-related outcomes (knowledge, attitudes, intentions, behaviour, service use).

Table 2.1 Research design and health promotion for young people: a mapping exercise

	Descriptive studies N (%)	Outcome evaluations N (%)	Total N (%)
Mental health	596 (94)	41 (6)	637 (100)
Healthy eating	259 (88)	36 (12)	295 (100)
Physical activity	323 (88)	45 (12)	368 (100)
Alcohol use/abuse	427 (87)	64 (13)	491 (100)
Illicit drugs	338 (91)	35 (9)	373 (100)
Tobacco	566 (73)	195 (27)	761 (100)
Total	2,509 (86)	416 (14)	2,925 (100)

Source: Peersman (1996).

Of the 2,925 references shown in Table 2.1, 86 per cent were descriptive studies; the range by topic was from 73 per cent (tobacco) to 94 per cent (mental health). The conclusion to the report of this mapping exercise was that those who want answers to the question 'what works in health promotion?' are faced with many obstacles, including how to find the primary studies, the fact that most research either does not report interventions or does not report evaluations, basic information about research design and methods is often missing and the conclusions presented by authors are frequently unreliable. 'Narrative reviews' which devote a paragraph to each of numerous intervention programmes describing different strategies, target populations, outcome measures, intensities and implementations leave the reader confused, and it is impossible to draw generalizable conclusions about the effectiveness of the approaches being studied.

Finding needles in haystacks (but not looking for gold)

Literature surveys of this kind are valuable in informing us about the extent and range of evaluation that has been done. However, more is needed to answer the question as to what is *trustworthy* about the conclusions that might be reached about the value of different approaches. This is particularly important for those who have to decide which health promotion initiatives to implement, and who may later have to defend their choice against counter-charges about weak evidence of doing more good than harm and/or at high cost.

It does work, doesn't it?

One relevant example is the current fashion for peer-delivered health promotion. As a generic concept, peer education has its roots in the monitorial system of British schools in the 1800s, in which, as a cost-saving exercise, teachers taught older students to teach younger ones. Peer education became popular for other reasons in the 1960s, when the notion of students being taught by their peers fitted with an ideological shift towards student-centred and experiential learning (Simons 1987). Peer education has also been vigorously promoted in the health promotion field, where it has been widely hailed as an effective approach (Aggleton 1997). There are many studies of peer-led health promotion, and many of these do claim that the approach works. Two examples, with their evaluation design, are described briefly below.

Peer sex education in schools in south-west England
(Phelps et al. 1994)

In 1992–3, 66 school students aged 16–17 years in south-west England were given two and a half days' training to discuss sexuality, sexual relationships, cultural pressure and resistance strategies with 38 secondary school classes of 13–14-year-olds in four weekly sessions. Of 900 students exposed to the peer programme, 336 answered pre-intervention questionnaires and 332 completed these afterwards. The questionnaires were anonymous, so pre- and post-data could not be matched for individuals. Differences between the questionnaire answers were analysed for evidence of the effectiveness of the peer lessons. Answers to three 'yes–no' questions about whether most teenagers have had sex by 16, and whether a girl can get pregnant the first time or during her period, showed increases of 8–33 per cent in correct answers. It was concluded that 'Evaluation illustrated that both the pupils and the peer leaders benefited from the programme' (Phelps *et al.* 1994: 138).

Drama education for prevention of alcohol abuse among teenagers in Canada (Walpole-Szabo and Sanagan 1987)

Three schools in Ontario took part in this study. Two schools hosted five theatrical 'skits' showing teenagers using and abusing alcohol; in one of these the skits were followed by peer-led discussion groups. The third school received no intervention. 'Approximately 450' students took part in the study, and were given before and after questionnaires; these were anonymous but carried birthdates to allow for matching, which was possible for 289 students. On three out of six scales measured in the questionnaires there was no apparent change in the experimental schools after either intervention, while on the other three there was a 'significant' interaction with school status (experimental or control), although in two the change was 'not that large'. The authors concluded that 'peer education benefits students' knowledge, attitudes, motivation and behaviour regarding the use of alcohol' and that a 'mandatory curriculum for alcohol education be developed using the concept of peer education' (Walpole-Szabo and Sanagan 1987: 170).

The question here concerns the relationship between the conclusions drawn by researchers and the data presented. Another way to phrase this question is to ask whether the authors have taken the trouble to rule out competing explanations. For example, in the first study, 63 per cent of the students offered peer education did not provide any information either before or after (or if they did this is not drawn on in the report). What might they have said, and how might this have affected the study's overall conclusions? Young people's understanding of, and knowledge about, sex and sexuality change over time. Might this have accounted for the apparent increase in knowledge which followed from the peer programme? Alternatively, could the findings be owing to different young people completing questionnaires after the intervention from those who provided information before it? The findings in the second study are based on data which omit the experiences of 36 per cent of the students who took part. While this study has a comparison group of students at a school which was not given either intervention, this school could have been very different in its student population, so the comparison might have been fairly pointless. In neither study does the analysis allow for the fact that students within schools, and even more so within the same classes, tend to be more alike in their backgrounds, attitudes and knowledge than students in different schools or classes. In short, it seems that the basis is somewhat thin in either study for claiming that peer education works. Any apparently positive effects of either intervention could well have been explained by other factors, and the evidence presented by authors is equally compatible with concluding that both interventions were ineffective or harmful.

Trying to be systematic

Systematic reviews are done in order to remedy the piecemeal picture which is gleaned from many such studies, and to draw on a much wider universe of knowledge. The two interventions described above represent fewer than 1 per cent of those found in a recent systematic review of the effectiveness and appropriateness of peer-delivered health promotion interventions for young people (Harden *et al.* 1999). This review found a total of 5,124 references to studies of peer education for young people (Table 2.2). These were located by searching five commercially available and six 'in-house'

Table 2.2   A systematic review of peer health promotion for young people

Total citations found	5,124
Met inclusion criteria*	**421**
Background studies (e.g. needs assessment, survey, review)	105
Reports of intervention studies	**316**
Non-evaluated interventions	62
Evaluated interventions	254
Evaluative reports of separate interventions	**210**
Outcome evaluations	133
Process evaluations	77
Met inclusion criteria*	130
Outcome evaluations	92
Process evaluations	38
'Sound' outcome evaluations	12
'Sound' process evaluations	2

* Interventions delivered by peers in a primary prevention of disease/health promotion context for young people aged 11–24 years; not peer counselling or using video, theatre or newsletters as primary medium of intervention; report available in English and hard copy obtainable within review time scale.
Source: Harden *et al.* (1999).

electronic databases (the years searched varied according to the database; see Harden *et al.* 1999 for details), and handsearching seven journals for the years 1996–8. Accessing non-commercial databases and handsearching found over a third of the studies. The large total of 5,124 references was narrowed down to 421 studies which met particular criteria (see Table 2.2). Out of the 421, 316 were reports of different types of peer health promotion intervention. Most of these were carried out in educational settings and used information only or skill development interventions deployed by young people of the same age or no more than a year older than the target group (although some 'peers' were quite a lot older).

Sixty-two (20 per cent) of the 316 intervention studies reported interventions without any accompanying evaluation. The review then went on to look in more detail at the 254 studies which also reported an evaluation. Some papers reported the same intervention (e.g. a longer-term follow-up, or a process evaluation of the same intervention described in a separate report from the outcome evaluation); in all there were 210 evaluative reports of separate interventions. These had been evaluated in 133 studies examining health promotion outcomes, and 77 reporting processes involved in implementing peer health promotion (57 of the 133 outcome studies also included process evaluations).

In further reviewing the quality of the outcome evaluations, the peer health promotion review used principles commonly accepted in health care evaluation for sorting out well designed from poorly designed intervention evaluations (Schwarz *et al.* 1980; Schaps *et al.* 1981; Loevinsohn 1990). A key issue, as can be seen from the above two examples of peer education, is the need to assess what happens to people who are exposed to a health promotion initiative against the standard of what might have happened had they not been exposed to it. The idea of a comparison group is simply to provide a means of understanding what might have happened without the intervention. In order to do this effectively, the comparison group needs to be made up of people who share similar characteristics with those receiving the intervention. If they do not do so, then any differences between them following the intervention may be due to pre-existing inequalities. Tossing a coin or randomization has been shown to be the most efficient method for creating unbiased comparison groups; there is otherwise nothing special about it (Kleijnen *et al.* 1997). Of course, random allocation does not, on its own, guarantee a well designed study. Other components of this are informed consent for all research participants, their involvement (or that of the 'target' community more generally) in designing the research tools, the collection of pre-intervention information on study outcomes and procedures for tapping and including in the analysis the experiences of all those who took part in the study.

Reading the outcome evaluations in the light of four methodological criteria – equivalent intervention and comparison groups, reporting of pre- and post-intervention data, and including information on all outcomes targeted – left the authors of the peer education review with 12 'sound' studies. In four of these there was evidence that peer health promotion was effective, in seven evidence of effectiveness for some outcomes and not others, while in the remaining study no evidence of effectiveness could be found.

This kind of research synthesis process puts the claims of the two studies described above, together with those of many others, in a somewhat different light. The relatively small number of studies which can be considered to provide reliable findings is the type of 'needle in a haystack' phenomenon that has been found across a whole range of social intervention topics (Oakley and Fullerton 1996).

Evaluating qualitative data

Some of the studies in the peer health promotion review combined data and evaluation designs from both sides of the 'paradigm war'. As noted above, intervention studies looking at outcomes can answer questions about effectiveness, provided they are designed appropriately, but other kinds of approaches are needed to answer other questions. It is perfectly possible to combine a range of questions in the same research design. For example, three ongoing studies of daycare for preschool children, support for socially disadvantaged families and peer-led sex education at secondary school level are all using the design of an RCT but are also including needs assessment, qualitative interviews, observations and user involvement in implementation and analysis issues to arrive at as full a picture as possible of what works and how it does (or does not) (Roberts et al. 1997; Stephenson et al. 1997; Oakley et al. 1998). In the daycare study, observations of children and staff in the study daycare centre are being combined with staff and parent interviews to give a fuller picture of the nature of the intervention and what it means to those involved. The social support and family health study is also using interviews with participants and with providers of the two interventions being tested (community support and supportive health visiting) to find out more about the experience of being researched and the social context in which the trial is being undertaken. Both trials include an economic evaluation, which will assess the costs and benefits of the interventions using a range of data. Chapter 10 illustrates how these processes of combining methods are working in the sex education trial.

There is, however, no doubt that much progress remains to be made in the field of health promotion evaluation in terms of combining different evaluation approaches. For example, in the peer health promotion review, only 8 per cent of the interventions in the outcome evaluation studies were based on data collected from young people about their own health promotion needs, and 55 per cent of these studies lacked any element of partnership with young people in implementing or evaluating the intervention. These gaps are potentially serious, since they make it more likely that interventions are not appropriate to the problems and circumstances for which they are designed, and are therefore liable to be ineffective and a waste of researchers', participants', and funders' time and money.

'Qualitative' approaches to evaluation cannot on their own guarantee trustworthiness. Similar issues of reliability to those asked of experimental data apply, with the key question being the extent to which researchers have taken steps to rule out the operation of bias in the collecting, reporting or analysis of research data. The process evaluations located for the peer health promotion review which reported a formative, intermediate or summative evaluation (i.e. evaluations at the start, midpoint or end of an intervention looking at implementation issues) were read to see whether they met commonly proposed standards for qualitative research (see, for example, Cobb and Hagemaster 1987; Boulton *et al.* 1996; Medical Sociology Group 1996; Popay *et al.* 1998): an explicit rationale for conducting the study; clear statement of aims, context, sample and methodology; analysis of data by more than one researcher; and inclusion of sufficient original data to allow readers to link evidence and interpretation. While most of the studies stated their aims clearly (73 per cent), offered a clear description of context (67 per cent) and included sufficient original data (67 per cent), fewer than half (47 per cent) stated an explicit framework in terms of theory or a literature review and just over half (53 per cent) offered a clear description of the sample, and in only 20 per cent of the studies were the data analysed by more than one researcher. At the end of this review process, only two of the process evaluations met all seven criteria and thus could be considered 'sound'.

It may be argued that these criteria are too demanding, or that the attempt to describe 'qualitative' research in the same terms as quantitative research is in itself misguided. But when it comes to hard questions about which health promotion initiatives to encourage and fund, the question of effectiveness in improving people's lives must surely be an extremely important one. Table 2.3 shows how claims to effectiveness are related to evaluation design in a different field, that of workplace health promotion. Estimates of effectiveness are considerably higher in outcome evaluations which lack control groups (some of which use 'qualitative' methods to examine effectiveness) than with well designed experimental studies.

Conclusion: future challenges

How evaluations are done is related to *what* they find: it is because of the relationship between the 'how' and the 'what' that debating evaluation design in health promotion is more than an 'academic' issue. The shift in thinking outlined in Chapter 1 about underlying features of health promotion

Table 2.3   Workplace health promotion interventions aimed at reducing cholesterol level

	Effective interventions according to authors (%)
All studies (N = 52)	81
Studies with no control group* (N = 22)	95
All trials (N = 30)	70
Well designed trials[†] (N = 12)	58

* Including those which used 'qualitative' methods to examine effectiveness
[†] Comparable intervention and comparison groups, pre- and post-intervention data, reporting on all outcomes
Source: Peersman et al. (1999).

as a 'postmodern' enterprise has been accompanied by a hardening of the warfare between 'quantitative'/experimental and 'qualitative' research methods. But all professionals have a duty to do more good than harm, and in this sense the ethical responsibility of health promotion practitioners and decision-makers is exactly the same as it is in medicine. Indeed, it has been argued that addressing questions of effectiveness through reliable evaluation designs is even *more* important in health promotion than in health care, because the people exposed to health promotion interventions are generally not sick in the first place (McCormick 1996). Health promotion can do harm as well as good; or it may have no effect, despite costing substantial amounts of money. These are all good reasons why well designed outcome evaluations need to have a key place in health promotion research. This does not, of course, mean that other types of research are not relevant, or, indeed, essential for answering other critical questions. What is important is that we leave behind the killing fields of the paradigm war and enter the more humane and kinder territory of combining methods and approaches in order to answer focused questions about how health promotion initiatives can enhance the quality and quantity of people's lives.

References

Aggleton, P. (1997) Health education: Vancouver Conference review. *AIDS Care*, 9(1), 35–9.

Bain, R. (1931) Behavioristic technique in sociological research. *Proceedings of the American Sociological Society*, 36, 155–64.

Beattie, A. (1997) Evaluation in community development for health: an opportunity for dialogue. In M. Sidell, L. Jones, J. Katz and A. Peberdy (eds) *Debates and Dilemmas in Promoting Health: A Reader*. Basingstoke: Macmillan.

Boruch, R. F. (1997) *Randomized Experiments for Planning and Evaluation*. Thousand Oaks, CA: Sage Publications.

Boruch, R. F. and Riecken, H. W. (eds) (1975) *Experimental Testing of Public Policy*. Boulder, CO: Westview Press.

Boulton, M., Fitzpatrick, R. and Swinburn, C. (1996) Qualitative research in health care II: a structured review and evaluation of studies. *Journal of Evaluation in Clinical Practice*, 2(3), 171–9.

Bryman, A. (1988) *Quantity and Quality in Social Research*. London: Unwin Hyman.

Bulmer, M. (ed.) (1984) *Sociological Research Methods: An Introduction*. Basingstoke: Macmillan.

Bunton, R. and Macdonald, G. (1992) Introduction. In R. Bunton and G. Macdonald (eds) *Health Promotion: Discipline and Diversity*. London: Routledge.

Campbell, D. T. and Stanley, J. C. (1963) *Experimental and Quasi-experimental Designs for Research*. Boston: Houghton-Mifflin.

Carr-Hill, R. (1995) Welcome? To the brave new world of evidence based medicine. *Social Science and Medicine*, 41(11), 1467–8.

Chalmers, I., Sackett, D. and Silagy, C. (1997) The Cochrane Collaboration. In A. Maynard and I. Chalmers (eds) *Non-random Reflections on Health Services Research*. London: BMJ Publishing Group.

Chapin, F. S. (1947) *Experimental Designs in Sociological Research*. New York: Harper and Row.

Cobb, A. K. and Hagemaster, J. N. (1987) Ten criteria for evaluating qualitative research proposals. *Journal of Nursing Education*, 26(4), 138–43.

Coyle, S. L., Boruch, R. F. and Turner, C. F. (1991) *Evaluating AIDS Prevention Programs*. Washington, DC: National Academy Press.

Davies, J. K. and Macdonald, G. (1998) Beyond uncertainty: leading health promotion into the twenty first century. In J. Macdonald and G. Davies (eds) *Quality, Evidence and Effectiveness in Health Promotion*. London: Routledge.

de Ven, P. and Aggleton, P. (1999) What constitutes evidence in HIV/AIDS education? *Health Education Research*, 14(4), 461–71.

Downie, R. S., Tannahill, C. and Tannahill, A. (1996) *Health Promotion: Models and Values*. Oxford: Oxford University Press.

Ferber, R. and Hirsch, W. Z. (1982) *Social Experimentation and Economic Policy*. Cambridge: Cambridge University Press.

Glass, G. V., McGaw, B. and Smith, M. L. (1981) *Meta-analysis in Social Research*. Beverly Hills, CA: Sage Publications.

Goodare, H. and Lockwood, S. (1999) Involving patients in clinical research (editorial). *British Medical Journal*, 319, 724–5.

Green, L. W. and Kreuter, M. W. (1991) *Health Promotion Planning: An Educational and Environmental Approach*. Toronto: Mayfield Publishing Company.

Greenwood, E. (1945) *Experimental Sociology*. New York: Octagon Books (reprinted 1976).

Hacking, I. (1990) *The Taming of Chance*. Cambridge: Cambridge University Press.

Harden, A., Weston, R. and Oakley, A. (1999) *A Review of the Effectiveness and Appropriateness of Peer-delivered Health Promotion Interventions for Young People*. London: EPI-Centre, Social Science Research Unit.

Hunt, M. (1997) *How Science Takes Stock: The Story of Meta-analysis*. New York: Russell Sage Foundation.

Kleijnen, J., Gotzsche, P., Kunz, R. A., Oxman, A. and Chalmers, I. (1997) So what's so special about randomisation? In A. Maynard and I. Chalmers (eds) *Non-random Reflections on Health Services Research*. London: BMJ Publishing Group.

Light, R. J. and Smith, P. V. (1971) Accumulating evidence: procedures for resolving contradictions among different research studies. *Harvard Educational Review*, 41(4), 429–71.

Loevinsohn, B. P. (1990) Health education interventions in developing countries: a methodological review of published articles. *International Journal of Epidemiology*, 4, 788–4.

Lundberg, G. (1933) Is sociology too scientific? *Sociologus*, 9 (September), 298–323.

McCall, W. A. (1923) *How to Experiment in Education*. New York: Macmillan.

McCormick, J. (1996) Medical hubris and the public health: the ethical dimension. *Journal of Clinical Epidemiology*, 49, 619–21.

McLaughlin, M. W. (1975) *Evaluation and Reform: The Elementary and Secondary Education Act of 1965*. Cambridge, MA: Ballinger.

Maynard, A. and Chalmers, I. (eds) (1997) *Non-random Reflections on Health Services Research*. London: BMJ Publishing Group.

Medical Sociology Group (1996) Criteria for the evaluation of qualitative research papers. *Medical Sociology News*, 22(1), 69–71.

Miller, J. L. and Lewis, M. (eds) (1987) *Research in Social Problems and Public Policy*. Greenwich, CT: JAI Press.

Nathan, R. P. (1988) *Social Science in Government*. New York: Basic Books.

Oakley, A. (1999) Paradigm wars: some thoughts on a personal and public trajectory. *International Journal of Social Research Methodology*, 2(3), 247–54.

Oakley, A. (2000) *Experiments in Knowing: Gender and Method in the Social Sciences*. Cambridge: Polity Press.

Oakley, A. and Fullerton, D. (1996) The lamppost of research: support or illumination? In A. Oakley and H. Roberts (eds) *Evaluating Social Interventions*. Ilford: Barnardos.

Oakley, A., Roberts, I., Mugford, M. and Barker, M. (1998) A randomised controlled trial and economic evaluation of two alternative strategies for providing support to socially disadvantged inner city families with infants. Unpublished protocol, Health Technology Assessment Programme.

Oliver, S. (1999) Users of health services: following their agenda. In S. Hood, B. Mayall and S. Oliver (eds) *Critical Issues in Social Research: Power and Prejudice*. Buckingham: Open University Press.

Peberdy, A. (1997a) Evaluation in health promotion: why do it? In J. Katz and A. Peberdy (eds) *Promoting Health: Knowledge and Practice*. Basingstoke: Macmillan.

Peberdy, A. (1997b) Evaluating community action. In L. Jones and M. Sidell (eds) *The Challenge of Promoting Health: Exploration and Action*. Basingstoke: Macmillan.

Peersman, G. (1999) *A Descriptive Mapping of Health Promotion Studies in Young People*. London: EPI-Centre, Social Science Research Unit.

Peersman, G., Harden, A., Oliver, S. and Oakley, A. (1998) *Reviews of Effectiveness in Health Promotion*. London: EPI-Centre, Social Science Research Unit.

Phelps, F. A., Mellanby, A. R., Crichton, N. J. and Tripp, J. H. (1994) Sex education: the effect of a peer programme on pupils (aged 13–14 years) and their peer leaders. *Health Education Journal*, 53, 127–39.

Philips, C., Palfrey, C. and Thomas, P. (1994) *Evaluating Health and Social Care.* London: Macmillan.

Popay, J., Rogers, A. and Williams, G. (1998) Rationale and standards for the systematic review of qualitative literature in health services research. *Qualitative Health Research*, 8(3), 341–51.

Roberts, I., Oakley, A. and Laing, G. (1997) Effects of out-of-home daycare on the health and welfare of socially disadvantaged families with children: a randomised controlled trial. Unpublished protocol, Department of Health.

Schaps, E., de Bartolo, R., Moskowitz, J., Pally, C. S. and Churgin, S. (1981) A review of 127 drug abuse prevention program evaluations. *Journal of Drug Issues*, 11(1), 17–43.

Schwarz, D., Flamant, R. and Lellouch, J. (1980) *Clinical Trials.* London: Academic Press.

Scott, S. (1992) Evaluation may change your life, but it won't solve all your problems. In P. Aggleton, P. Young, D. Moody, M. Kapila and M. Pye (eds) *Does It Work? Perspectives in the Evaluation of HIV/AIDS Health Promotion.* London: Health Education Authority.

Silverman, D. (1985) *Qualitative Methodology and Sociology.* Aldershot: Gower Press.

Simons, H. (1987) *Getting to Know Schools in a Democracy: The Politics and Process of Evaluation.* Brighton: Falmer Press.

Stephenson, J., Oakley, A., Johnson, A. and Brodala, A. (1997) A randomised intervention trial of peer-led sex education. Unpublished protocol, Medical Research Council.

Stevenson, H. M. and Burke, M. (1991) Bureaucratic logic in new social movement clothing: the limits of health promotion research. *Health Promotion International*, 6(4), 281–9.

Tones, K. (1997) Beyond the randomized control trial: a case for 'judicial review' (editorial). *Health Education Research*, 12, i–iv.

Turner, C. F., Miller, H. G. and Moses, L. E. (eds) (1989) *AIDS: Sexual Behavior and Intravenous Drug Use.* Washington, DC: National Academy Press.

Walpole-Szabo, G. and Sanagan, P. (1987) 'Booze' and today's teenager. *Canadian Journal of Public Health*, 78 (May/June), 168–70.

Williams, G. and Popay, J. (1997) Social science and the future of population health research. In L. Jones and M. Sidell (eds) *The Challenge of Promoting Health: Exploration and Action.* Basingstoke: Macmillan.

▶ **3**

▷ Learning from research

▷ **Greet Peersman and Ann Oakley**

Research as a source of information

A quality health promotion service should be right for the situation, fair and acceptable to everyone involved, should improve health and be value for money. If such claims are justifiable, it is an evidence-based health promotion service. Alternatively, if such claims are based on opinion rather than evidence they attract criticism, face difficulties with securing funding and provoke arguments about the best way forward. Claims may be justified, or refuted, by doing research: that is, developing and testing health promotion in such a way as to learn from the experience. Sometimes, a quicker route is to learn from others' experience, through reading research that is already completed.

Research reports may come from colleagues, be found through searching bibliographic databases, be seen when skimming journals or be circulated through departments or professional bodies. They may hold a reader's interest because they discuss innovative ideas for assessing needs or providing services; because they describe services that look promising and address a major health burden which is a local priority, with methods and resources that could fit the local strategy; or because they show services to be effective and ethically and principally sound. If they do none of these things they deserve rejection. Thus, familiarity with local services and circumstances guides readers' decisions about whether to consider the conclusions of a research report. Critical appraisal skills are also required to judge whether a report offers reliable conclusions about the effectiveness of an intervention (see Chapter 6). This chapter discusses the problems service providers face when attempting to use research to guide service planning and describes the major lines of work of the EPPI-Centre in aiming to address some of these issues. It sets the scene for other chapters in this book which take these issues up in more detail.

Challenges in using research

An American national survey of 284 HIV prevention programme managers found that most of them do not turn to research, nor do they perceive it as an important source of information. Peers and colleagues topped the list of information sources influencing programme decisions; scientific publications ranked at the very bottom, along with government and other non-academic reports and mainstream newspapers (Goldstein *et al.* 1998). It is quite possible that interactions with peers and colleagues include discussions of research and therefore it cannot be concluded that research is *not* being used. Nevertheless, scientific publications seem to play a rather insignificant role. Factors prohibiting programme managers from identifying research as an important and useful resource in programme planning included the perception that information does not exist (for example, that research has not been conducted on the topic or population of interest), the time it takes to find and the cost of accessing relevant research reports. They also indicated that information needed not only to be readily available – for example, on-line or as clippings, summaries or other compilations – but also to use language that is familiar to service providers (Goldstein *et al.* 1998). Similar problems were reported by health promotion purchasers and providers in the UK (see Chapter 11).

In addition to the lack of efficient access to health promotion research in terms of both locating research and language, the quality of reporting is often low. In a review of 112 outcome evaluation studies of sexual health promotion interventions for young people (Peersman *et al.* 1996), 15 per cent of studies did not include an abstract, the majority of studies (63 per cent) failed to report the social class background and nearly 30 per cent did not provide any details on the ethnic composition of the study population. In as many as 67 per cent of the studies, the theoretical basis for the intervention was absent or not indicated. Issues of consent were not reported in more than half the studies (55 per cent) and details of the outcomes targeted by the intervention were absent from 5 per cent. In 33 (30 per cent) of the studies, the length of the interval for follow-up evaluation was not specified, and 17 (15 per cent) failed to report the impact on all outcomes targeted. The lack of clear reporting seriously reduces the potential contribution research can make to informed decision-making. These examples are certainly not unique. They bring up important issues that need to be addressed if research is to be used more routinely for improving services.

Clearly, increasing the use of research requires multiple strategies at multiple levels. Some issues need to be addressed when funding research, such as considering how useful research will be to service delivery, and planning the dissemination of research findings. Increasing the funding of research of interest to local users is one strategy. To establish local research priorities, a research advisory group may be established including local service providers and users, as well as programme managers and policy makers. This group can also work together with researchers on the design of the study and assist in problem-solving throughout the course of the study (Richardson *et al.* 1990). Soliciting comments about the usefulness of research from referees at the proposal stage of a study is another means of addressing expected use. Plans for disseminating research findings can be made in advance of awarding research grants. Indeed, grant-awarding bodies may wish to develop and resource their own dissemination strategy, or at least require grant proposals to include an explicit and comprehensive dissemination procedure.

Researchers themselves can play an important role in facilitating the use of their research. For example, to ensure that the information needs of 'customers' are likely to be met, researchers can: discuss the kinds of research products that will be aimed for and how they can be used, at the outset of the study; be explicit in their research reports about the aims of the research, the study design and methods and the implications of the research findings, including any shortcomings; participate in informal meetings with potential users of the research findings, to ensure a clear understanding of the research reports; or assist with the translation of research findings using language that is appropriate to a range of audiences (Richardson *et al.* 1990). How some of this has been done to support the preparation of a systematic review is recorded in Chapter 8.

Increasing access to research

A great deal of health promotion research has been conducted, but only some is in the public domain and, overall, its literature is widely dispersed. Access through electronic databases, such as Medline and EMBASE, may appear quick, but these are rather clumsy tools for locating health promotion studies. Searching is often labour-intensive, especially if getting a good overview of the available research is the aim (see Chapter 4). For example, the EPPI-Centre aimed to find *well designed* outcome evaluations in a range of health promotion areas, including sexual health promotion for young people, workplace health promotion and accident prevention for older people. Within the limited time frame available for the work, we were able to acquire 781 (60 per cent) full reports of the outcome evaluation studies identified. Of these, 309 (40 per cent) described an RCT, 237 (30 per cent) a non-randomized trial and 235 (30 per cent) used another evaluation design. But only 16 (5 per cent) of the 309 reports of an RCT included the term 'RCT' or 'randomized trial' in the title; an additional six (2 per cent) used 'controlled trial'; 52 (17 per cent) mentioned at least 'trial'. Of the 93 RCTs identified from electronic databases, two (11 per cent) of the 18 RCTs identified from Medline lacked the specific Medline Publication Type tag 'RCT'; of the 21 RCTs identified from EMBASE, only four (19 per cent) had 'RCT' as an EMBASE descriptor, and nine (43 per cent; including the four RCT-labelled studies) had the specific EMBASE tag 'controlled study'. The 54 RCTs identified from other electronic databases (Aidsline, ERIC, HealthPromis, PsycLIT, Social Science Citation Index) did not have specific RCT tags. This means that health promotion specialists turning to commercial databases for RCTs are likely to be misled into thinking that there are few, if any, RCTs available that are relevant to their work.

As part of its continuing programme of work in conducting literature reviews in health promotion, the EPPI-Centre has carried out a variety of systematic searches over the years (see also Chapter 4). A systematic search involves using explicit, well documented search strategies and employing a wide range of search methods, including electronic databases, finding additional references from citations of research reports, conducting thorough handsearches of key journals in the field and contacting major research institutions and research funders. The results of these searches were compiled into a database using ProCite, commercially available software for managing references. We refer to this bibliographic register as BiblioMap. Rather than relying on the wide variety of terms that were used for indexing the references on the different electronic databases from which they originated – mostly medical or educational – or the keywords which are often part of the summary or abstract of a journal paper, we developed a standardized coding strategy. This offered two major advantages. First, the coding could be applied consistently to all reports irrespective of their origin, hence making the retrieval of references from BiblioMap very efficient. Second, terminology was chosen specifically to reflect that of the health promotion field.

The resulting systematic coding strategy (Peersman and Oliver 1997) aimed to classify the studies according to their design, the country where they were carried out, their health topic area and the basic socio-demographic characteristics of their study population. In addition, reports of intervention studies were also coded for the programme name (e.g. Smokebusters, Stop AIDS), the intervention site, the intervention provider and the type of intervention. Where a study reported an evaluation of the impact of an intervention on health outcomes, details of the evaluation design were also coded. The EPPI-Centre team collected as many full reports as possible of identified references in the area of health promotion for young people, a continuing task. Subsequently, a team of ten postgraduate research students and experienced researchers were trained in the systematic coding procedures and tackled the coding of the reports obtained. When full reports were not yet obtained, coding was based on the information available, usually an abstract or summary. All coding was then entered on BiblioMap. Currently, this regularly updated register contains approximately 8,000 references which can be searched by author, title and any combination of the associated standardized coding; of these, 6,820 are fully coded to date. For example, using the search terms 'process evaluation' and 'workplace site' retrieves references relevant to answer the question: 'How can we work with employers to improve the health of employees?' Another practical question is, for example, 'Can we combine healthy eating and tobacco control in an effective intervention delivered in the primary care setting?' Relevant references can be retrieved by using 'outcome evaluation' and 'healthy eating' and 'tobacco' and 'primary care'. Or 'how many health promotion interventions have included legislation as a vehicle for behaviour change?' can be answered by using the search term 'legislation' to indicate the type of intervention. Over the years, the EPPI-Centre has provided researchers, health promotion providers and policy makers with lists of bibliographic references specific to their area of interest. Thus, BiblioMap provides an efficient short-cut to identifying specific types of health promotion studies, which are otherwise obtained through rather cumbersome methods, or missed altogether.

Mapping research activity

Because BiblioMap is the result of systematic and comprehensive searching for research reports within the field of health promotion, it is also a tool that can be used for the 'descriptive mapping' of this field; in other words, for describing the focus and extent of health promotion research. This also identifies research gaps which allows a cost-efficient and timely allocation of resources for future research. For example, of the total of 6,820 fully coded references classified according to the type of study, we found that the majority (4,331; 63 per cent) were descriptive studies (i.e. case–control studies, cohort studies, reviews, systematic reviews, meta-analyses). A total of 1,497 (22 per cent) were reports of the evaluation of health promotion interventions, of which 1,293 (86 per cent) included the examination of knowledge, attitude and/or behavioural outcomes (i.e. were outcome evaluations). Only 222 (15 per cent) of the 1,497 evaluative studies included both process and outcome measures; and only 44 (3 per cent) included an economic evaluation or any indication of costs associated with the intervention. These results show how small a proportion of both the health promotion field in general, and the evaluation field in particular, is directly relevant to the question of 'what works?' In addition, the impact of many interventions has been assessed on intermediate outcomes rather than on health outcomes *per se*. These issues may be addressed in two different ways: by commissioning more rigorous evaluation research that includes a wide range of process as well as outcome measures and, at the same time, by ensuring that the findings from evaluation studies are more likely to make it into the public domain, a problem already discussed above.

Another example of how descriptive mapping may be used is the assessment of the extent to which current thinking in health promotion practice is reflected in the available research. In the past decades, the discourse around health promotion practice has shifted from a focus on individual lifestyles to full and organized community participation and self-reliance (see Chapter 1). Good health promotion interventions are considered to be those that are addressing a problem that has been identified as a priority issue by the community itself, and that are involving the community in the development and delivery of interventions that are targeted at different settings (e.g. school, workplace, community) simultaneously (Ziglio 1996). Of the 1,293 outcome evaluations of health promotion interventions mentioned above, only 2 per cent were carried out in developing countries; and very few (2 per cent) focused on reducing health inequalities by specifically targeting disadvantaged populations in so-called resource-rich countries. The vast majority (80 per cent) of studies involved populations in institutionalized settings (formal education, health care system, workplace); few (14 per cent) took place in a community setting and even fewer (3 per cent) by means of outreach. Only 17 per cent tackled particular health problems concurrently in different settings. These figures are problematic in the sense that although socially disadvantaged groups and countries should be specifically targeted to tackle health inequalities, most health promotion research has been carried out in well resourced countries and with easy-to-reach populations. For example, more than 90 per cent of people with HIV live in developing countries but most of the research capacity is located in the established market economies. There is an urgent need to bridge this gap through the development of prevention programmes that are evaluated within the local context, and through increasing access to health care in general.

Although the boundaries between different settings are artificial as far as people's health and its determinants are concerned, few interventions have tackled health issues across settings. It is important, for example, that young people receive consistent messages about smoking in school, at home and in the community. Very often, though, parents of teenagers are smokers themselves, and laws prohibiting the sale of tobacco products to teenagers are not always enforced. It is clear that a concerted health promotion effort is needed to tackle smoking in young people. In addition, it is well known that the majority of disadvantaged populations worldwide live in circumstances that offer little intersection with formal education, health services or the workplace setting; and most of them live in situations that make them especially vulnerable to health and other problems. Hence, more effort and resources need to be expended on community-based and outreach activities. In terms of the types of interventions provided, 25 per cent included education only, 22 per cent aimed at increasing access to resources and/or services, 9 per cent involved an environmental modification and regulation (such as a smoking ban) or legislation (such as a cycle helmet law) were the subject of only 5 per cent of intervention studies. The majority (65 per cent) of interventions were individualized approaches; only 26 per cent provided an individualized approach complemented by at least one change in the environment to support behaviour change. Despite the fact that increased knowledge rarely in itself produces behaviour change or the ability to increase control over one's health, a quarter of interventions consisted of education only. Interventions addressing the wider social context were limited in both frequency and scope. The results from this comprehensive descriptive mapping exercise seem to indicate a rather unbalanced research portfolio in health promotion.

Reviews of research

Although BiblioMap describes research activity, it does not record valid research findings. Important questions remain, such as 'What is the methodological status of evaluation research in health promotion?' and 'How much evidence do we have about the impact of health promotion interventions on health?' One of the important questions, as noted above, is 'Does it work?' Finding an answer to this question is an essential step in setting priorities for action and in allocating resources. Typically, reviews of effectiveness have attempted to address this question. They aim to synthesize findings from different individual studies that have focused on a common health problem and that have evaluated the effect of health promotion interventions on health-related outcomes. Examples of such reviews are: 'The impact of incentives and competitions on participation and quit rates in worksite smoking cessation programs' (Matson et al. 1993); 'The effectiveness of sexual health interventions for young people' (Peersman et al. 1996); 'Dental caries in developing countries in relation to the appropriate use of fluoride' (Manji and Fejerskov 1990). Over the past few years, there has been increasing enthusiasm for undertaking effectiveness reviews in different areas of health promotion. As a result of a systematic search, the EPPI-Centre identified 398 completed and 39 ongoing effectiveness reviews. Of these, 39 per cent were reviews related to the impact of substance abuse (drug, alcohol, tobacco) interventions, and 18 per cent were effectiveness reviews within the sexual health field; all other areas of health promotion were covered to a lesser extent (typically fewer than 10 per cent of the reviews covered areas of injury prevention, healthy eating, mental health etc.). A significant feature of all this review activity has been the lack of a central register listing the reviews being conducted. This has led to a situation in which concurrent reviews have often overlapped in the questions they address, and the primary studies they examine. However, the search strategies used for identifying relevant studies, the criteria for including studies and the methods for combining results from different studies have been distinctly different. Research has shown that using different review methods may alter the conclusions about effectiveness, and hence the knowledge to guide implementation about effective interventions (Peersman *et al.* 1999a, b). Consequently, what is 'known' about what works in health promotion is heavily dependent on 'what questions' have been asked and 'how' they have been addressed.

In order to describe the review methods used (see also Chapters 6 and 7) in the above identified 398 effectiveness reviews, reporting on the following was assessed: the purpose of the review; the methods used for identifying primary studies; criteria used for inclusion of studies; and criteria used for assessing the validity of primary research. It was also noted how the findings were presented. The results showed that a quarter of the reviews failed to state the purpose for the review, i.e. did not provide a frame of reference helping the reader to decide whether to read on, or setting a scope for determining strategies in the selection of primary studies. Only a third of the reviews (33 per cent) reported their search strategy, and even fewer provided it in sufficient detail for it to be replicated. This makes it very difficult for the reader to assess whether the range of included studies does represent the existing knowledge base in a particular area, or whether it is likely that relevant materials have been missed. Fewer than a third of reviews (27 per cent) indicated the criteria by which the methodological quality of the included studies was assessed, though 66 per cent of reviews included some weighting of the included studies (i.e. discussed at least to a certain extent the strengths and weaknesses of the design and execution of at least *some* of the studies). Very few reviews (16 per cent) included both a narrative synthesis and a formal meta-analysis, i.e. a statistical pooling of the findings from different studies; most reviews provided a narrative synthesis only. Fewer than half (42 per cent) of the reviews presented a summary table of all included primary research. Only 75 reviews (19 per cent) reported *all* of the following: aims, search strategy, inclusion criteria and validity criteria. Why are these findings problematic? Overall, the lack of clarity in review methodology implies that it is fairly difficult, if not impossible, to assess the potential bias and hence the reliability of most of the available effectiveness reviews, though the vast majority (81 per cent) of these reviews made recommendations for services and/or directions for future research. Nevertheless, reviews – whatever their methods – provide an important short-cut to finding primary studies in different areas of health promotion. A searchable register of literature reviews identified by the EPPI-Centre is available on the Web (http://eppi.ioe.ac.uk/).

EPPI-Centre reviews

Wider recognition of the key role of reviews in synthesizing and disseminating the results of effectiveness research has prompted people to consider their validity. 'Systematic' reviews differ from other types of reviews in that they use explicit, systematic methods with the aim of limiting bias (systematic errors) and reducing random errors, thus providing more reliable results upon which to draw conclusions and make decisions (Mulrow and Oxman 1997) (see also Chapter 7 and 8). Rather than reflecting the views of the authors, or a restricted selection of the available literature, systematic reviews provide a more comprehensive summary of what we know and do not know about different forms of health care interventions (Deeks et al. 1996). Systematic reviews establish where the effects of health care are consistent, allowing research results to be applied across populations, settings and differences in intervention; and where effects may vary significantly. As such, they are important tools for service providers and policy makers to guide programme planning and implementation. In addition, by identifying areas of knowledge and gaps in knowledge, they are also an invaluable first step before carrying out new primary research.

In order to answer questions about effectiveness systematically, the EPPI-Centre developed a standardized approach (Peersman et al. 1997) to collating data from primary studies focused on the planning, content, delivery and implementation of the intervention, the study population, the design and findings of the outcome evaluation and, if available, the characteristics and findings of the associated process evaluation. The aim was to integrate systematically qualitative and quantitative research about interventions and their impact, and to include information on cost where available. An assessment of the methodological rigour of the studies is included but all studies in a particular area of health promotion are described in detail irrespective of the study design. However, for the purpose of recommendations for policy, practice and future research, only the findings from methodologically rigorous studies are relied upon (see Chapter 7).

Bibliographic information and descriptive data, as well as evaluation findings, are then compiled on EPIC, a database developed in-house. This database allows for the user-friendly retrieval of effectiveness data by health topic area, study population, setting, approach and a range of other parameters, such as different outcome measures. For example, in answer to the question 'what types of school-based sexual health promotion interventions have a positive effect on health-related outcomes?', seven studies were retrieved from EPIC. In addition to being able to look at the detail of each individual study, EPIC allows for an overview and further analysis of the studies in terms of their key characteristics (see Table 3.1). Shared characteristics, if any, of effective interventions can then be compared with those of interventions that have failed to work. The latter studies can be pulled and analysed from EPIC in a similar fashion. In this way, questions that are specific to local concerns may be answered directly, provided research studies are available in that area of interest.

The EPPI-Centre has provided: tailored information on the effectiveness of health promotion interventions, using EPIC; guidance in developing

Table 3.1 Effectiveness database, EPIC: what works in secondary schools?

Detail of interest	Effective studies	
Country	USA	6
	Sweden	1
Type of intervention	Information/education	5
	Practical skills	3
Intervention provider	Health promotion practitioner	1
	Researcher	2
	Teacher	3
Medium of intervention	Curriculum materials	6
	Discussion groups	5
	Practising skills	2
	Presentation/lecture	4
	Printed materials/posters	2
	Role play	2
	Theatre/film/video	1
Length of intervention	One day to one week	2
	One week to one month	2
	Up to two years	1
Outcomes	Attitudes	5
	Awareness/beliefs	2
	Behaviour	2
	Intentions	2
	Knowledge	7
	Self-efficacy	1

Note: N = 7.

systematic search strategies; training in critical appraisal skills and systematic reviewing; and assistance in the design of evaluation studies. Several EPPI-Centre reports of systematic reviews of effectiveness of health promotion interventions have also been produced (France-Dawson *et al.* 1994; Holland *et al.* 1994; Oakley and Fullerton 1994, 1995; Oakley *et al.* 1994a, b, 1995a, b, c, 1996).

The above examples demonstrate how BiblioMap and EPIC can be used to provide more efficient and direct access to research reports that can answer questions of local concern. A range of other specialist databases have also been compiled by others in the field, and these are discussed in more detail in Chapters 4 and 7. Now that research is increasingly available, health promotion practitioners can adapt their working practices to accommodate it. Considerable progress has been made to date to facilitate the use of research, but a lot more needs to be done than just enhancing access to research findings. A pertinent question is 'To what extent *can* research influence prevention practice?' Implementing evidence-based interventions requires changes in the way professionals work as well as in the way organizations operate. Though this is challenging at times, there are many successful examples (see Chapters 8, 10 and 12) of how researchers, service providers and users can work together to improve health promotion services and, ultimately, health.

References

Deeks, J., Glanville, J. and Sheldon, T. (1996) *Undertaking Systematic Reviews of Research on Effectiveness. CRD Guidelines for Those Carrying out or Commissioning Reviews.* York: NHS Centre for Reviews and Dissemination, University of York.

France-Dawson, M., Holland, J., Fullerton, D. *et al.* (1994) *Review of Effectiveness of Workplace Health Promotion Interventions.* London: Social Science Research Unit. (Updated in G. Peersman, A. Harden and S. Oliver (1998) *Review of Effectiveness of Health Promotion Interventions in the Workplace.* London: Health Education Authority.)

Goldstein, E., Wrubel, J., Faigeles, B. and DeCarlo, P. (1998) Sources of information for HIV prevention program managers: a national survey. *AIDS Education and Prevention*, 10(1), 63–74.

Holland, J., Arnold, S., Fullerton, D., Oakley, A. and Hart, G. (1994) *Review of Effectiveness of Health Promotion Interventions for Men who Have Sex with Men.* London: Social Science Research Unit. (Updated in A. Oakley, S. Oliver, G. Peersman and M. Mauthner (1996) *Review of Effectiveness of Health Promotion Interventions for Men who Have Sex with Men.* London: EPI-Centre, Social Science Research Unit.)

Manji, F. and Fejerskov, O. (1990) Dental caries in developing countries in relation to the appropriate use of fluoride. *Journal of Dental Research*, 69, 733–41.

Matson, D., Lee, J. and Hopp, J. (1993) The impact of incentives and competitions on participation and quit rates in worksite smoking cessation programs. *American Journal of Health Promotion*, 7(4), 270–80.

Mulrow, C. and Oxman, A. (1997) *How to Conduct a Cochrane Systematic Review.* San Antonio: Cochrane Collaboration.

Oakley, A., France-Dawson, M., Fullerton, D. *et al.* (1995a) *Review of Effectiveness of Health Promotion Interventions to Prevent Accidents in Older People.* London: Social Science Research Unit.

Oakley, A., France-Dawson, M., Fullerton, D. *et al.* (1996) Preventing falls and subsequent injury in older people. *Effective Health Care*, 2(4), 1–16.

Oakley, A. and Fullerton, D. (1994) *Risk, Knowledge and Behaviour: HIV/AIDS Education Programmes and Young People.* London: Social Science Research Unit.

Oakley, A. and Fullerton, D. (1995) *Young People and Smoking.* London: Social Science Research Unit.

Oakley, A., Fullerton, D. and Holland, J. (1995b) Behavioural interventions for HIV/AIDS prevention. *AIDS*, 9, 449–86.

Oakley, A., Fullerton, D., Holland, J. *et al.* (1994a) *Reviews of Effectiveness: HIV Prevention and Sexual Health Education Interventions.* London: Social Science Research Unit.

Oakley, A., Fullerton, D., Holland, J. *et al.* (1994b) *Reviews of Effectiveness: Sexual Health Interventions for Young People*. London: Social Science Research Unit. (Updated in G. Peersman, A. Oakley, S. Oliver and J. Thomas (1996) *Review of effectiveness of sexual health promotion interventions for young people*. London: EPI-Centre, Social Science Research Unit.)

Oakley, A., Fullerton, D., Holland, J. *et al.* (1995c) Sexual health education interventions for young people: a methodological review. *British Medical Journal*, 310, 158–62.

Peersman, G., Harden, A., Oliver, S. and Oakley, A. (1999a) *Effectiveness Reviews in Health Promotion*. London: EPI-Centre, Social Science Research Unit.

Peersman, G., Harden, A., Oliver, S. and Oakley, A. (1999b) Discrepancies in findings from effectiveness reviews: the case of health promotion interventions to change cholesterol levels. *Health Education Journal*, 58, 192–202.

Peersman, G., Oakley, A., Oliver, S. and Thomas, J. (1996) *Review of Effectiveness of Sexual Health Promotion Interventions for Young People*. London: EPI-Centre, Social Science Research Unit.

Peersman, G. and Oliver, S. (1997) *Keywording Strategy. Data Collection for the BiblioMap Database*. London: EPI-Centre, Social Science Research Unit.

Peersman, G., Oliver, S. and Oakley, A. (1997) *EPI-Centre Review Guidelines. Data Collection for the EPIC Database*. London: EPI-Centre, Social Science Research Unit.

Richardson, A., Jackson, C. and Sykes, W. (1990) *Taking Research Seriously. Means of Improving and Accessing the Use and Dissemination of Research*. London: HMSO.

Ziglio, E. (1996) How to move towards evidence-based health promotion interventions. Paper presented at the Third European Conference on effectiveness and quality assessment in health promotion and health education, Turin, Italy, 12–14 September.

▶ **Part 2**

▷ Finding and appraising research
evidence

▶ 4

▷ Finding research evidence: systematic searching

▷ **Angela Harden**

Using relevant research that is already completed is quicker and cheaper than mounting new studies. Finding that research is the challenge. What you find and how much depends on how you approach searching the literature. A hastily constructed search of the most easily accessible database may leave you either overwhelmed by the vast number of references retrieved or disappointed by the apparent lack of relevant research. This chapter aims to provide a problem-based account of seeking research systematically to answer practical questions within health promotion.

What is systematic searching?

A common theme running throughout the chapter is the value of *systematic* searching methods. A search that is systematic is thoughtfully planned, carefully executed and accurately recorded. The aim is to find relevant research whether it is readily available or difficult to access. Systematic search methods are also explicit and transparent; they are open to scrutiny and available for repeating or extending. By contrast, *unsystematic* searching is haphazardly planned and executed, can lead to a partial or distorted picture of the research literature in a particular area and is incompletely recorded or not recorded at all. Whether quick or comprehensive, a search which is systematic will be more productive. Using two contrasting searching tasks as examples, the following sections take you step-by-step through the searching process.

Two hypothetical searching tasks[1]

Task one is for a health promotion specialist, based in the health promotion department of a local health authority. He[2] is looking for ideas to develop an effective resource for local schools to promote sexual health. He has three to four months to do this and will only realistically have a few days over the space of two to three weeks for planning and conducting a search.

Task two involves a policy maker from a large union organization developing national policy guidelines about health promotion for the workforce. She needs to find out whether workplace health promotion benefits employees and employers or not (or, indeed, whether it is harmful) and which kinds of programmes should be recommended. She has one to two months available for searching and has a researcher or an information scientist working alongside her to undertake the searching.

What type of research is needed?

Being clear about what research is needed is a prerequisite for designing a search strategy. The task may demand that research is focused on a particular *health topic* (e.g. cardiovascular disease, drugs), *population group* (e.g. young people, smokers), health promotion *setting* (e.g. workplace, school), *type* of health promotion (e.g. legislation, tailored advice, skill development, providing access to resources, community development, partnerships) or *provider* of health promotion (e.g. health professional, psychologist, teacher). The health promotion focus may be very general (e.g. promoting health in community settings) or quite specific (e.g. using peers to promote sexual health for young people in secondary schools). Whatever the interest, defining the *health promotion focus* is an essential first step.

The second step is to be clear about the question needing an answer. Is the task about determining health promotion needs or how to recognize them? For instance, what are the health concerns of a particular community and what are the important factors which need to be targeted by health promotion initiatives? Or is the question about what works? Perhaps the question of interest is about how interventions work or about factors that may influence local implementation of an intervention. Perhaps all such questions are of interest. Because different study designs answer different research questions, it is worth identifying the type of question the research is needed to answer and then specifying what *type of research design* it needs to be able to answer the question.

Considering the two tasks described above in terms of the *health promotion focus* and the *type of research design* will help to inform the choice of particular sources to search and how to search them, and will help to evaluate the search results. Even if the intention is to recruit the services of a skilled librarian, this process will help to explain the searching task to them. Table 4.1 shows how the two searching tasks have been translated into search questions with their health promotion focus and the type of research specified.

Table 4.1 Translation of two hypothetical tasks into search questions, health promotion focus and type of research required

Aim of task	Searching task(s)	Health promotion focus			Type of research study
		Health topic	Setting	Population	
Task 1: To develop a resource for local schools on promoting sexual health	To find research answering the following questions: 1 What resources have been shown to be effective in schools? 2 What do young people see as important in promoting their sexual health? 3 How can these resources be used in local schools?	Pregnancy prevention; STD prevention; promotion of positive sexual relationships	Secondary education	Young people aged 11–16	1 Outcome evaluations 2 Process evaluations 3 Process evaluations
Task 2: To develop national policy guidelines on the benefit of health promotion programmes in the workplace	To find research answering the following question: is health promotion provided in the workplace effective in improving the health of the workforce?	Various topics	Workplace	Adults	Outcome evaluations

In terms of health promotion focus, task one requires research focused on pregnancy prevention or STD prevention or upon broader sexual health issues such as the promotion of positive sexual relationships. To develop the resource, information will be needed from a variety of research types: research which has examined the effectiveness of resources (provided by outcome evaluations); details on the views of young people themselves on sexual health promotion (provided by process evaluations); and guidance on the best ways to implement such strategies (also provided by process evaluations). In contrast, task two requires research focused on various health topics set in the workplace. It is primarily focused on locating research that examines whether health promotion programmes are effective (i.e. outcome evaluations).

So how might the health promotion specialist and the policy maker approach their searching tasks given the different resources they have available to them?

A quick search to find an effective resource

Bearing in mind that the health promotion specialist only needs to find one effective resource applicable to local schools for promoting sexual health to complete his task, he has a number of options that might prove productive.

Visiting a library

Perhaps the most obvious way to find research is to walk into any university library and flick through any books or journals which appear relevant. After telling the librarian his searching task, the health promotion specialist learns that although there do not yet exist any journals specifically concerned with promoting sexual health, the library subscribes to one journal that is concerned with the treatment and prevention of STDs (*Sexually Transmitted Diseases*) and several journals that are devoted to health promotion/education and public health in general which may contain specific articles on promoting sexual health (e.g. *Health Education Research: Theory and Practice* and *Health Promotion International*). As the health promotion specialist only has a couple of hours to spare, he decides to look through the issues of each journal for the past two years only (1999–2000). He doesn't find any relevant articles in *Sexually Transmitted Diseases*. Although some of the articles in this journal were about preventing STDs, most prevention efforts were set in STD clinics and none were in schools. However, he finds five relevant articles from *Health Education Research* and one from *Health Promotion International*. These can be photocopied at the library to be read and critically appraised (see Chapter 6) before using their key messages in preparing the resource.

There are thus several advantages to this method of searching: quick access to relevant research; help from a librarian in choosing which journals to search; judgements about the relevance of a piece of research can be made on the full report rather than on the abstract and/or title only; and any article deemed relevant can be photocopied there and then and taken away. However, this approach will miss relevant articles in other journals or issues. What is found is highly selective and not representative of all the research in this area. In addition, the number of relevant articles found may not justify the time taken. The health promotion specialist looked through a total of 44 issues with a total of 420 articles across the three journals to find the five reports of relevant research.

Professional contacts

Asking someone who knows can be a quick way to find something relevant. Beyond immediate colleagues, the first port of call should be national bodies with a remit for health promotion (e.g. the Health Development Agency in England) or other health promotion units. These may be able to identify relevant research themselves or identify other organizations to contact. A further method is to make use of already existing professional networks and relevant email discussion lists. Concerning the latter, there are several which are relevant to health promotion and public health (for a full list and details of how to sign up see http://www.mailbase.co.uk and http://www.jismail.ac.uk/default.htm). Contacting professional networks and organizations is likely to unearth practitioner research which can be particularly valuable in guiding the development and delivery of interventions.

Systematic reviews of effectiveness

To complement reports about these practical aspects, this task needs information about effectiveness. A short-cut to effectiveness information is provided by systematic reviews which attempt to find as much as possible of all the research literature available within the area of interest (see Chapter 7 for more details). As the number of systematic reviews is increasing, several sources have become available for locating these reviews. The majority are freely accessible via the Web. These sources can be divided into two main types: those which provide searchable databases of systematic reviews conducted by many different agencies and those which are the websites of specific agencies listing the reviews conducted by that agency.

Two general sources of systematic reviews are the Cochrane Database of Systematic Reviews and the Database of Reviews of Effectiveness (DARE). Cochrane reviews are generally considered to be very rigorous and all reviews on DARE are quality assessed. Both of these can be searched simultaneously on the Cochrane Library, which gives access to the full reports of Cochrane reviews. The health promotion specialist starts his search by using the MeSH term 'sex education'. ('MeSH terms', or Medical Subject Headings, is how the Cochrane Database and DARE keyword reviews according to topics. See below under 'Bibliographic databases' for more information.) This doesn't bring up any systematic reviews in the Cochrane Database but a summary and the bibliographic details for two systematic reviews are found on DARE.

He then tries the EPPI-Centre's register of reviews (http://eppi.ioe.ac.uk). For searching this database he selects the terms 'sexual health', 'pregnancy prevention' or 'std' and combines them with the term 'young people'. For potentially high-quality reviews, he limits the search to only those which possess all the methodological quality attributes which the reviews are coded for (see Chapter 7 for a discussion of quality in systematic reviews). He finds a total of seven citations to five separate relevant systematic reviews, six of which are relevant to school-based sexual health promotion. Of these two had already been found on DARE, giving him a total of six relevant systematic reviews. These included reviews specifically about school-based sex education (e.g. Stout and Rivara 1989), while others were not exclusively focused on school-based interventions (e.g. Peersman *et al.* 1996a).

Bibliographic databases

If our busy practitioner wishes to broaden his search he can turn to bibliographic databases, which are electronic catalogues for storing research that has been published primarily in academic and practice journals. There are two main types of bibliographic databases: 'general' databases, which aim to catalogue as much as possible of all research within a particular discipline or area, usually run by commercial organizations; and 'specialist' registers compiled for a much narrower topic area or for a much more specific purpose. Although each database differs in its scope, comprehensiveness, access and searching facilities (see Table 4.2 for details), common to all is the basic 'unit' of the database: the bibliographic citation (as shown in Figure 4.1). Usually, but certainly not always, the citation comes with an abstract summarizing the research and its findings and a set of terms which classify the research according to certain areas. Following the abstract in the example in Figure 4.1 (not shown in full) is a long list of words taken from the 'controlled vocabulary' or 'keywords' of the database in which the citation was found (in this case MEDLINE). The controlled vocabulary is a standardized list of terms used to describe the content of the research reports. As resources are limited, he decides to use MEDLINE, which is the only 'general' database freely accessible over the Internet, and two specialist registers. The first is HealthPromis from the Health Development Agency (England). The second is BiblioMap, the specialist register of the EPPI-Centre.

Authors, year of publication, title, source

Schou, L. and Wight, C. (1994) Does dental health education affect inequalities in dental health? Community.Dental Health. 11(2):97-100.

Abstract The aim of the study was to evaluate the Lothian 1991 dental health campaigns on 5-year-old schoolchildren's oral hygiene and gingival health in relation to deprivation. A stratified random sample of 486 children was selected from 92 primary schools in the city of Edinburgh. Clinical examinations took place immediately before (T1), a month after (T2) and 4 months after the campaign (T3) . . . .

Child, Preschool; Comparative Study; Dental Plaque/*prevention & control; Dental Plaque Index; Female; Gingival Diseases/*prevention & control; *Health Education, Dental; Human; Knowledge, Attitudes, Practice; Male; Oral Hygiene/education/*statistics & numerical data; Oral Hygiene Index; Periodontal Index; Poverty; Program Evaluation; Psychosocial Deprivation; School Dentistry; Scotland; *Social Class

Controlled vocabulary/keywords

Figure 4.1 The bibliographic citation
Source: taken from MEDLINE.

Starting with the smaller specialist databases, he searches HealthPromis first, using the database's controlled vocabulary, known as the 'Thesaurus'. There is a thesaurus term for sex education so he decides to use this combined with the free-text term 'school'. This gives him a total of 38 references.

He then turns to BiblioMap, the specialist register held at the EPPI-Centre. The controlled vocabulary used by BiblioMap has two special features: it uses a flexible, but comparatively short, list of terms to code research according to health promotion focus; and it codes all studies according to the type of research design it uses. He asks EPPI-Centre staff to search for process evaluations of sexual health promotion conducted in secondary schools in the UK. To do this the staff combine the keywords 'process evaluation' with the terms 'sexual health' or 'pregnancy prevention' or 'STD' and the term 'secondary education'. This gives a total of 63 citations.

Going on to search MEDLINE, a large general database of bibliographic references, he types in the term 'sex education' as a (good) guess on what might generate citations of relevant research. This brings up 4,374 references. A quick scan of the first ten of these reveals that there are only one or two which look really relevant. As he tries to work out why this search has brought up so many irrelevant citations (e.g. one on the clinical manifestation of Alzheimer's disease), he realizes that typing in 'sex education' has

Table 4.2 Summary of sources of research evidence

Source	Scope	Access details	How to search	Advantages/disadvantages
Quality assessed and synthesized research evidence				
Examples of searchable databases				
The Cochrane Database of Systematic Reviews	All areas of health care; systematic reviews.	By subscription to the Cochrane Library for access to full reviews; bibliographic details searchable via the NHS Centre for Reviews and Dissemination (University of York) website (see below).	Using MeSH terms from MEDLINE or 'free-text'. Relevant terms for health promotion include 'health-promotion', 'health-education', 'primary-prevention', 'preventative-health-services'.	• Evidence in the reviews is already critically appraised and synthesized. • Some provide access to the full review (Cochrane Library and DARE). • All reviews meet a minimum standard of quality (Cochrane Library and DARE) or those of a higher quality are easily identifiable (EPPI-Centre Register of Reviews of Effectiveness). • Controlled vocabulary of Cochrane Library and DARE rely on Medical Subject Headings (MeSH), which may make it more difficult to find reviews relevant to health promotion/public health.
Database of Reviews of Effectiveness (DARE)	All areas of health care; systematic reviews.	Searchable via the NHS Centre for Reviews and Dissemination (University of York) website: http://agatha.york.ac.uk	Using MeSH terms from MEDLINE (e.g. 'Health-Promotion', 'HIV-Prevention') or 'free-text'. For terms relevant to health promotion see above.	
The EPPI-Centre Register of Reviews of Effectiveness in Health Promotion	Health promotion/public health focus; systematic and non-systematic reviews.	http://eppi.ioe.ac.uk	Using a health promotion specific controlled vocabulary. Each entry is coded according to topic area (e.g. accidents, healthy eating), population group (e.g. young people, children), type of review (e.g. systematic review, meta-analysis) and methodological attributes of review (e.g. methods of searching given).	

Examples of the websites of agencies which have carried out systematic reviews

Agency	Focus	URL	How to find	Notes
Public Health Effectiveness Project	Health promotion/public health focus; systematic reviews.	http://www.health.hamilton-went.on.ca/CSARB/EPHPP/ephpp.htm	By scanning the titles of completed reviews/summaries of reviews.	• EPPI-Centre Register of Reviews of Effectiveness is specific to health promotion and uses health promotion specific controlled vocabulary for easy retrieval.
Health Development Agency	Health promotion/public health focus; systematic reviews.	http://www.hda-online.org.uk/indicators.htm	By scanning the titles of completed reviews/summaries of reviews.	• Evidence in the reviews is already critically appraised and synthesized.
Health Evidence Bulletins – Wales	Health care in general; systematic reviews.	http://www.uwcm.ac.uk/uwcm/lb/pep/index.html	By scanning the titles of completed reviews/summaries of reviews.	• Access to full review available on some sites.
Health Technology Assessment (HTA) monographs	Health care in general; systematic reviews.	http://www.nhsweb.nhs.uk/	By scanning the titles of completed reviews/summaries of reviews.	• Some sites are not health promotion specific (HTA and Health Evidence Bulletins – Wales).

Table 4.2 (cont'd)

Source	Scope	Access details	How to search	Advantages/disadvantages
Bibliographic databases				
Commercially available				
MEDLINE	Primarily a medical database, but contains citations relevant to health care from a range of social sciences.	http://www.ncbi.nlm.nih.gov/	Using MeSH terms or free-text terms. For terms relevant to health promotion, see above. Searches can be limited to randomized controlled trials only.	• Catalogue a huge amount of research. • Exhaustive searches require considerable skill and knowledge. • Do not generally provide access to full papers. • Research found is not critically appraised. • Limited to published research only. • Bias towards research published in the English language (although EMBASE has better coverage of European journals than MEDLINE).
EMBASE	Primarily a medical database, but contains citations relevant to health care from a range of social sciences.	By subscription only.	Using a set controlled vocabulary known as 'Medical Descriptors' or free-text terms. Relevant terms for health promotion include 'health promotion', 'health education', 'primary prevention', 'education program'.	
PsycLIT	Catalogues the psychological research literature.	By subscription only.	Using a psychological controlled vocabulary. Relevant terms for health promotion include 'health education', 'primary mental health promotion', 'preventive medicine', 'health behavior'.	

Social Science Citation Index	All social sciences (e.g. psychology, sociology, economics, political science).	By subscription only.	Using free-text terms only.	
ERIC	Catalogues the educational research literature.	By subscription only.	Using an educational controlled vocabulary. Relevant terms for health promotion include 'health education', 'health promotion', 'health programs', 'preventive medicine', 'behavior change'.	

Specialized registers

HealthPromis (provided by the Health Promotion Information Centre (HpiC) of the Health Development Agency, England)	Health promotion specific; catalogues research as well as other resources (e.g. videos, pamphlets, websites). Currently contains 52,000 records.	http://healthpromis.hea.org.uk/	Using free-text or the HPiC Thesaurus (based on the 'Multi-lingual European Thesaurus on Health Promotion).	• Health promotion specific (except for CCTR), which can make them less time consuming to search more accurately. • May not be as comprehensive as commercially available databases, but may be better sources of unpublished and 'grey' literature. • Do not generally provide access to full papers.
Health Promotion Library Scotland (HPLS) (provided by Health Education Board Scotland)	Health promotion specific; catalogues research from over 350 journals as well as other resources (e.g. books, pamphlets).	http://www.hebs.scot.nhs.uk/researchcentre/glib/index.htm	Using free-text or searching on keywords relevant to health promotion.	

Table 4.2 (cont'd)

Source	Scope	Access details	How to search	Advantages/disadvantages
BiblioMap (provided by the EPPI-Centre, Social Science Research Unit, University of London, Institute of Education)	Health promotion specific; most comprehensive for all types of research with young people (currently approx. 8,000 entires).	Currently through contacting EPPI-Centre staff: health@ioe.ac.uk	Using free-text or a controlled vocabulary. Each record is coded according to type of research, country, health focus and population, and, for studies evaluating or describing an intervention, intervention site, provider and type.	• Research found is not critically appraised. • BiblioMap and CCTR specifically developed to facilitate evidence-based health promotion. It is therefore easier to find research according to specific research design/ methods.
The Cochrane Controlled Trials Register (CCTR) (Provided through the Cochrane Library)	Health care in general; main focus on randomized controlled trials (currently approx. 800 are relevant to health promotion).	By subscription only, but can be accessed via the Cochrane Health Promotion Field (contact health@ioe.ac.uk)	Using free-text or MeSH terms. For examples of terms relevant to health promotion see above.	

This table does not attempt to be a comprehensive listing of all sources of research relevant to health promotion but does try to give a comprehensive range of examples.

The EPPI-Centre and the NHS Centre for Reviews and Dissemination (University of York) also have searchable websites available of the reviews which these agencies have carried out. In some cases, access to the full review is available via these websites.

brought up: all citations in which the terms 'sex' and 'education' appear consecutively anywhere in the bibliographic citation regardless of whether the research is actually about sex education; citations which have the term 'sex education' in the abstract but which have as a main focus another topic; citations which are about adults rather than young people; and citations which refer to research conducted in settings other than schools. In other words, he has got a real 'mixed bag'. He tries a few different terms, such as 'sex education in schools', which retrieves 535 citations, 'educating young people about sex', which retrieves 54 citations, and 'promoting young people's sexual health', which brings up 18 citations. These do bring up more relevant records in numbers that the health promotion specialist can handle and he may want to stop his search here. However, if he does, he needs to accept that he will only have found a fraction of what may be potentially useful to him. What the health promotion specialist is using here is a searching technique called 'free-text searching'. This technique, while essential in some circumstances, can be an inaccurate way to search.

A more precise way to search is to use the controlled vocabulary of a database. For MEDLINE this vocabulary is known as 'MeSH' (Medical Subject Headings). Accessing MeSH terms using the 'MeSH Browser', he finds that there is a 'MeSH' term for 'sex education'. Searching using this term brings up 3,918 references, but scanning the first ten he realizes that this time many more of them seem to be at least of some relevance. He still finds he has retrieved citations which are about adults rather than young people so he needs to find the subset which are about school-based sex education. Again using the MeSH browser he finds the MeSH term 'school'. The next stage is to put these controlled vocabulary terms together in a 'search string'. He wants to find citations which have been assigned the MeSH term 'sex education' *and* the MeSH term 'schools'. The technical language that will enable him to search in this way is the 'Boolean' operator 'AND', used between the two terms. This reduces his set of references to 282, a more manageable number to deal with. A way of recording the completed search along with the results is demonstrated in Table 4.3.

Table 4.3   Development of a search strategy on MEDLINE

	Search string	Result
Finding citations of research about sex education	#1 Sex education [MeSH Terms]	3,918
Finding citations of research set in schools	#2 Schools [MeSH Terms]	35,631
Finding citations of research about sex education in schools	#3 #1 AND #2	282

However, he wants to get an idea of how much of the relevant research which actually exists on HealthPromis or MEDLINE he has found, and does this by exploring the controlled vocabulary of each database in a lot more depth. He finds that there were many more terms he could have used to identify research relevant to sexual health on both MEDLINE (e.g. 'acquired immunodeficiency syndrome', 'condoms', 'contraception', 'contraception behavior') and HealthPromis (e.g. 'HIV/AIDS', 'sexual health', 'sexually transmitted diseases', 'unintended pregnancy', 'safer sex').

Although using controlled vocabulary terms was more helpful in identifying relevant reports on this occasion, there will be times when 'free-text' searching is essential (Reed and Baxter, 1994). This particularly applies to areas of health promotion that involve the use of new concepts or specialist terminology for which controlled vocabulary does not yet exist. For example, finding research on certain approaches, such as peer education, or research on tackling inequalities and the wider determinants of health, may require very creative use of 'free-text' searching. This is where specialist registers of research specific to health promotion may be valuable, as their controlled vocabulary is likely to represent much more accurately health promotion specific concepts and approaches.

He now has 320 citations from MEDLINE and specialist registers together (some citations appeared on two or more of them). He scans the citations and finds a total of 43 references which (on the basis of title and abstract) are relevant to his task.

The comprehensive search: is workplace health promotion effective?

Unlike the practitioner above, the union policy maker does not need, yet, information about development and delivery of an intervention. Instead she needs all effectiveness information about any health promotion interventions in the workplace.

Systematic reviews of effectiveness

The policy maker also decides to use these databases of systematic reviews. She does a free-text search using various combinations of 'workplace' for the Cochrane database and DARE and uses the keyword 'workplace' on the EPPI-Centre Register of Reviews of Effectiveness. She finds a total of 19 systematic reviews (six from DARE or the Cochrane Library and 16 from the EPPI-Centre, which means that three reviews were common to both databases) which are potentially of a good quality. Some of these are on workplace health promotion in general (e.g. Heaney and Goetzel 1997; Peersman et al. 1998), while others are focused on specific health topics such as preventing back injuries (Karas and Conrad 1996) or occupational health and safety (Goldenhar and Shulte 1994). However, as the searches for the most up-to-date review were conducted in 1997, she decides that it is worth finding more studies to make sure that her recommendations take into account the very latest available evidence.

Bibliographic databases

Relevant databases are likely to include commercially available ones such as MEDLINE, PsycLIT and the Social Science Citation Index, as well as specialized registers. Looking back at Table 4.1, the policy maker needs to find research: (a) that is focused on promoting health or preventing disease; (b) that is conducted in the workplace; and (c) that evaluates interventions in terms of their effectiveness. Again, the starting point in constructing a search strategy for each database is to identify terms in the database's controlled vocabulary which correspond to these three areas. The aim of this task is to find all relevant studies with an 'exhaustive' search. The policy maker already has around thirty studies in her filing cabinet which meet these three criteria. If she can find these on the database she is going to search, this will be a good way of finding the relevant controlled vocabulary terms to use to identify further studies. Table 4.4 shows the results of this exercise for the first four studies which are in the filing cabinets.

This technique is known as 'pearl growing' and involves using an initial number of relevant articles to 'grow' other ones. Table 4.4 highlights several important things which all have implications for how the policy maker needs to search to ensure that she increases her chances of finding as much as possible of all available research. First, not all databases catalogue all three studies. This suggests that the policy maker is right to decide to search more than one database. Second, the Social Science Citation Index does not use controlled vocabulary to describe studies. This means that, for this database, the policy maker will have to rely on 'free-text' searching. Third, each database has slightly different sets of controlled vocabulary. For example, MEDLINE uses the term 'Occupational Health Services' to indicate the workplace context of Kronenfeld *et al.* (1987), whereas PsycLIT uses 'Employee Assistance Programs'. So the policy maker needs to develop a search strategy for each database separately. Fourth, as in the sexual health searching example, more than one controlled vocabulary term is available to retrieve articles according to a particular criteria. For example, MEDLINE and PsycLIT both use the obvious term 'health promotion' to indicate that Glasgow *et al.* (1997) reports on research about health promotion, but they also use other, perhaps less explicit, terms (e.g. 'health behavior', 'knowledge attitudes practice', 'cardiovascular disease/prevention and control'). This indicates that the policy maker may have to use multiple terms to search under each of her search criteria. Finally, controlled vocabulary for each of the search criteria has not always been applied. For example,

Table 4.4 The controlled vocabulary used on three bibliographic databases to catalogue three studies examining the effectiveness of workplace health promotion

	MEDLINE	PsycLIT	Social Science Citation Index
Kronenfeld JJ, Jackson K, Blair SN, Davis K, Gimarc JD, Salisbury Z, Maysey D, & McGee JG. (1987). Evaluating Health Promotion: A Longitudinal Quasi-Experimental Design. *Health Education Quarterly*, 14(2), 123–139.	Health-Promotion; Occupational-Health-Services; Alcohol-Drinking; Diet-; Exertion-; Longitudinal-Studies; Seat-Belts; Smoking-prevention-and-control; South-Carolina; Stress-Psychological-prevention-and-control	Program-Evaluation; Health-Behavior; Employee-Assistance-Programs; Health-Education; Government-Personnel; Longitudinal-Studies	Not found
Glasgow, R; Terborg JR; Strycker LA; Boles, SM and Hollis JF Take heart II: Replication of a worksite health promotion trial. *Journal of Behavioral Medicine.* 1997; 20(2): 143–161.	Adult-; Aged-; Cohort studies; Comparative study; Coronary Disease/prevention and control, psychology; Cross-sectional studies; Female-; Health Behavior; Health Promotion; Human-; Hypercholesteroleminia/prevention and control, psychology; Knowledge, attitudes, practice; Life-style; Male-; Middle Age; Risk-factors; Treatment outcomes	Behavior-change; Eating-; Employee-Assistance-Programs; Health Promotion; Social-support-networks; Adulthood-; Cholesterol-; Health-behavior; Personnel-; Tobacco-; Smoking-	Not found
Guldan GS, Zhang Y, Huang Y, Yang X, & Zeng G. (1992). Effectiveness of a worksite education activity in a factory in China. *Asia-Pacific Journal of Public Health*, 6(2), 8–14.	Health-Education-methods; Knowledge,-Attitudes,-Practice; Nutrition-Education; Occupational-Health-Services; China-; Diet-; Food-; Metallurgy-; Teaching-methods	Not found	Not found
Jeffery RW, French SA, Raether C, Baxter JE (1994) An environmental intervention to increase fruit and salad purchases in a cafeteria, *Preventive Medicine*, 23, 788–92	Food-Preferences-psychology; Restaurants; Fruit-; Adult-	Health Promotion; Consumer-Behavior; Diets-; Eating-; Choice-Behavior; Costs-and-Cost-Analysis; Adulthood-	Found but no controlled vocabulary

MEDLINE is the only database to assign controlled vocabulary according to study design ('treatment outcome') to indicate that the research has evaluated an intervention according to effectiveness, and it does this for only one of the four studies found on MEDLINE (Glasgow *et al.* 1997). This is one of the major drawbacks of these databases and it is well documented that controlled vocabulary for study design is currently inadequate or too inconsistently applied to be very useful (Dickersin *et al.* 1995; Peersman *et al.* 1996b; Harden *et al.* 1999; Glanville and Lefebvre 2000). This suggests that there are no reliable means for the policy maker to limit her search to only research that evaluates effectiveness.

Using the results of this exercise combined with looking for more relevant controlled vocabulary in each database's thesaurus (for those which have one), and considering where 'free-text' terms are needed, she constructs a search strategy which will find as many as possible back from the ten studies she knows are on the databases. The final search strategy for PsycLIT is shown in Table 4.5.

Handsearching

When more resources are available and an exhaustive search is possible, handsearching, although labour-intensive, is crucial. No matter how comprehensive bibliographic databases or specialized registers claim to be, it is

Table 4.5 A search strategy for PsycLIT to locate research on workplace health promotion

Searching task	Search terms	
Finding citations of research relevant to health promotion/disease prevention	#1	Health Promotion [Thesaurus term]
	#2	Health Education [Thesaurus term]
	#3	#1 OR #2
Finding citations of research set in the workplace	#4	Employee Assistance Programs [Thesaurus term]
	#5	Personnel [Thesaurus term]
	#6	Workplace ['free-text']
	#7	Worksite ['free-text']
	#8	Employee ['free-text']
	#9	#4 OR #5 OR #6 OR #7 OR #8
Finding citation of research relevant to workplace health promotion	#10	#3 AND #9

For 'free-text' terms it will be important to use all variations of the term which could appear in the abstract or title of the bibliographic citation (e.g. 'workplace' could appear as 'workplaces', 'work place', 'work-place' etc.)

virtually impossible to find all the research that exists on a particular topic through these sources (Dickersin *et al.* 1995; Harden *et al.* 1999; Peersman *et al.* 1999).

As well as seeking some advice from a librarian on which journals to search (as outlined in the previous example), a further systematic way of choosing the journals which are likely to yield the most research is for her to examine the bibliographic citations of the relevant research which she has already identified. From this she can identify, say, the top five journals in which outcome evaluations of workplace health promotion are most frequently published. Another systematic way in which she could identify journals for handsearching would be to choose journals which are not covered by the bibliographic databases she has searched. For example, she may know that the journal *Occupational Medicine* is only indexed on MEDLINE, a database which she has not searched and does not intend to search.

Scanning reference lists

This source of research involves looking through the list of research that has been referred to ('cited') in relevant research which has already been identified, to identify further relevant pieces of research. Scanning reference lists, like personal contacts, can be very useful when little research has been identified or when an exhaustive search is essential. The main disadvantage, however, is that reference lists only provide details on the title of reports of research, so it might be quite difficult to tell if a particular citation is going to be relevant or not. Obtaining full reports can be a time consuming exercise (it involves identifying which library stocks the journal that the research is published in, going to that library, photocopying it etc.), so it may be a real waste of effort tracking down a piece of research and then not finding that it is relevant. For example, the policy maker scans the reference list of a piece of research she has already identified and finds what looks to be a further piece of relevant research reported in an article entitled 'Mobile worksite programs'. As it is published in a journal not available at her local library she has to order it on inter-library loan. After three weeks, it finally arrives. However, the article turns out not to be reporting on a piece of research, nor is it relevant to health promotion.

Professional contacts

Remembering that it is impossible to find all the research which exists in a particular area via bibliographic databases, contacting individuals may help in locating as much research as possible. Researchers with an interest in the area are most likely to know of relevant effectiveness studies, and their addresses can be found on their publications. Unfortunately, few reply to such enquiries.

Documenting and evaluating search results

Tips have been provided throughout this chapter on how to document the search strategy used and the results found. While such documentation can seem laborious, it helps to ensure that searching is done systematically and helps with evaluating the searching techniques and results. For evaluating the search, at least three interrelated questions need to be considered. Did the searching identify enough relevant research? How much effort was involved in finding the relevant research? Was the effort worth it? What constitutes 'enough' research is likely to vary depending on the searching task. For the health promotion practitioner, finding one good systematic review and enough process evaluations to illustrate the range of issues which need to be considered by schools in promoting sexual health may be enough. For the policy maker, on the other hand, 'enough' research is likely to mean finding as much as is possible. Part of the documentation of the search conducted for task one is shown in Table 4.6.

As shown in the last column, the health promotion specialist has found a total of 115 process evaluations of school-based sexual health promotion. He knows that his search will not have been exhaustive as he has not

Table 4.6   Documentation and search results for task one

General source of research	Specific source of research	Time taken/resources needed			Total citations found	Relevant citations found
		To develop search[b]	Scan through results[b]	Obtain full report[b]		
Personal contacts	Ten organizations (e.g. Health Development Agency)	Half a day to write letters	None	Papers and/ or citations obtained from five people up to a week later	4	4
Hand searching	44 issues across three journals searched	None	Equivalent to half a day's work	Full reports obtained immediately	5	5
Bibliographic databases[a]	HealthPromis	1 hr	30 mins	Waited for	36	15[c]
	BiblioMap	1 hr	30 mins	2–3 weeks	63	63
	MEDLINE	3–4 hrs	3–4 hrs	for all reports to be obtained	287	28[b]

[a] Searches carried out on 21 September 2000.
[b] These figures are based on informed estimates based on the experiences of EPPI-Centre staff in conducting and documenting searches within the area of sexual health promotion.
[c] This figure is based on the author scanning through the titles of the 36 citations to identify which ones could potentially be process evaluations.

searched all the bibliographic databases available and the search strategies he used on them were designed for ease rather than comprehensiveness; his handsearching of journals was 'opportunistic' (limited to relevant journals available in his local library); and he did not chase up personal contacts who did not respond to his requests. However, he can make this explicit in the resource he develops so that readers can judge for themselves the evidence on which it has been based. In terms of how much effort was required, it is clear that the most effort was associated with searching the bibliographic databases, but this source also provided the highest yield, which suggests that the effort was worth it. However, this may apply to HealthPromis and BiblioMap only as a larger proportion of what was identified on these databases actually turned out to be relevant (only 10 per cent of the citations identified on MEDLINE were relevant). For hand-searching and personal contacts all the pieces of research identified were relevant, but the effort to yield ratio was clearly higher. However, this may be offset by the fact that obtaining full reports of the research is imme-diate, at least for handsearching. This example shows how a number of factors have to be balanced against each other in the evaluation of a search strategy.

Conclusions

The examples used in this chapter suggest that lots of research is available to inform policy and practice for health promotion. Finding it is by no means an easy task but, taking a systematic approach, searching currently available resources can be extremely productive. Examining the advantages and disadvantages of different sources of research according to two differ-ent searching tasks has revealed a number of key messages:

- Clearly defining the health promotion focus and type of research needed for a particular task forms the basis for a systematic approach to searching.
- Considering the time and resources available determines which sources of research to search and how many.
- All sources of research evidence have limits to their comprehensiveness. Some may be more comprehensive than others for research according to topic area, disciplines covered, country in which the research was carried out, place and type of publication etc. Searching more than one source is, therefore, important.
- Searching sources of quality-assessed and synthesized research should always be the first port of call when looking for evidence of effectiveness.
- Developing productive search strategies for 'general' bibliographic data-bases can be complex. When resources are limited, searching 'specialist' databases may be more cost-effective.

- Knowledge of the scope and limitations of each source of evidence can make explicit any potential biases in search results.
- Accurately documenting the searching process is essential for evaluating search results and for making transparent to others how the search has been conducted.

Notes

1 These tasks represent just two examples of searches which practitioners, policy makers or researchers may undertake. While not based on real examples, the searching tasks and the resources available to complete them have been informed through the searching requests which EPPI-Centre staff receive through its information and enquiry service and through informal and formal discussions held with different professional groups involved in health promotion (e.g. Oliver *et al.* 1996).

2 For simplicity I have made the health promotion specialist male and the policy maker female. I am not, of course, assuming that all health promotion specialists are male and that all policy makers are female.

References

Dickersin, K., Scherer, R. and Lefebvre, C. (1995) Identifying relevant studies for systematic reviews. In I. Chalmers and D. Altman (eds) *Systematic Reviews*. London: BMJ Publishers.

Glanville, J. and Lefebvre, C. (2000) Identifying systematic reviews: key resources. *Evidence Based Medicine*, 5, 68–9.

Goldenhar, L. M. and Schulte, P. A. (1994) Intervention research in occupational health and safety. *Journal of Occupational Medicine*, 36(7), 763–75.

Harden, A., Peersman, G., Oliver, S. and Oakley, A. (1999) Identifying relevant primary research on electronic databases to inform decision-making in health promotion: the case of sexual health promotion. *Health Education Journal*, 58, 290–301.

Heaney, C. A. and Goetzel, R. Z. (1997) A review of health-related outcomes of multi-component worksite health promotion programs. *American Journal of Health Promotion*, 11(4), 290–307.

Karas, B. E. and Conrad, K. M. (1996) Back injury prevention interventions in the workplace: an integrative review. *American Association of Occupational Health Nurses*, 44(4), 189–96.

Oliver, S., Nicholas, A. and Oakley, A. (1996) *Promoting Health after Sifting the Evidence: Workshop Report*. London: EPI-Centre, Social Science Research Unit.

Peersman, G., Harden, A. and Oliver, S. (1998) *Effectiveness of Health Promotion Interventions in the Workplace: A Review*. London: Health Education Authority.

Peersman, G., Harden, A., Oliver, S. and Oakley, A. (1999) Effectiveness reviews in health promotion: different methods, different recommendations. *Health Education Journal*, 58, 192–202.

Peersman, G., Oakley, A., Oliver, S. and Thomas, J. (1996a) *Review of Effectiveness of Sexual Health Promotion Interventions for Young People.* London: EPI-Centre, Social Science Research Unit.

Peersman, G., Oakley, A. and Oliver, S. (1996b) Evidence-based health promotion? Some methodological challenges. *Health Promotion and Education,* 37(2), 59–64.

Reed, J. and Baxter, P. (1994) Using reference databases. In H. Cooper and L. Hedges (eds) *The Handbook of Research Synthesis.* New York: Russell Sage Foundation.

Stout, J. and Rivara, F. (1989) Schools sex education: does it work? *Pediatrics,* 83(3): 375–9.

▶ 5

▷ # World Wide Web for health: how to access tools and research

▷ **James Thomas**

There must be very few people in the UK who have not heard about the Internet and have not seen – at least on television – an Internet browser with a Web page being displayed. The popular media portrayal of the Internet as a high-tech business opportunity and the accompanying rush to encourage people to use on-line shopping facilities might, however, be obscuring one of the Internet's primary aims: that of making information accessible to a very wide audience. A large number of organizations with relevant information for health promotion researchers and practitioners are now using the Internet to disseminate their work. This should enable us to be more informed about current practices and debates than ever before, since the information is – quite literally – at our fingertips.

Accessible information is not necessarily reliable information. This chapter, therefore, has three main aims: in addition to introducing the Internet and the World Wide Web as useful tools for health promotion research, it raises a number of important issues to bear in mind when using the Internet and also describes ways in which the Internet can be used, both in conducting research and in locating the findings of research. (Experienced Internet users may wish to skim through the opening sections of this chapter to the section entitled 'Locating evidence on the Internet'.)

An introduction to the Internet

This part of the chapter introduces the Internet briefly: how it works, how to use it and some of the common terminology that has grown up around it.

The 'Internet' is the term used to describe the network of computers (and other devices) linked together across the world over cables and satellites in a way that enables information to be exchanged between each individual computer (or device). The Internet has been designed to work with a large number of different devices: PCs, Apple Macs and large mainframe computers share the same means of communication with mobile telephones and TV sets. This wide range of media has presented numerous challenges to programmers, since protocols for communication needed to be developed which could be understood by a very diverse range of devices. While a means of communication has been agreed, together with a mechanism for locating computers on the Internet, the actual computers found there are simply there because one person – or a group of people – decided that they wanted to place them there: usually in order to disseminate some information. There is no central body governing which information should and should not be published, and this is one reason why the Internet can appear to be very confusing and disorganized. Another reason – again because of the way the Internet evolved – is the number of ways of using it. Early users had to negotiate their way through a bewildering array of terms and acronyms: gopher, telnet, FTP, NSFNET, BITNET are just a few of them. The World Wide Web (WWW, W3 or 'the Web') is a relative newcomer to Internet terminology, but because of its visual content and (relative!) ease of use, it became the main means of using the Internet, and some of the older protocols have become obsolete. Like the rest of the Internet, the World Wide Web is a network of linked computers. It differs from other aspects of the Internet in the way that the files it holds (documents) are linked to one another, enabling users to move between them at the click of a mouse button (see below). The computers which hold these documents available for reading are known as *websites* or *web servers*.

The rate of growth of the Internet has also been a source of some of its problems. In June 1993 it was estimated that there were just 130 websites.[1] By June 2000 this number had grown to 17,119,262. This growth in websites has been mirrored by a similar growth in the number of people using them. Nua Internet Surveys[2] estimated that in July 2000 there were 359.8 million people on-line throughout the world. Some 19.47 million people (32.72 per cent of the population) in the UK were reported to be on-line in June 2000, up from 960,000 (2 per cent) in June 1997. However, this growth in access to the Internet has not been as 'worldwide' as might be thought. There is growing evidence of a 'digital divide' between countries which have invested heavily in Internet infrastructure and those which cannot afford to. There is a danger that countries which cannot take advantage of the opportunities offered by the Internet could be condemned to economic stagnation,[3] which would undoubtedly affect the health and education of their populations. This digital divide does not only operate on an international level. Research in the UK has shown that the Internet is reinforcing unequal social divisions,[4] and that the installation of Internet terminals in libraries and shopping centres does little to overcome this without accompanying training for novice users.[5]

Issues of accessibility also arise when the construction of websites is examined. Blind people navigate the Web using a speech synthesizer, and there are other specially developed devices to allow people with other disabilities to use the Web in other ways. Sites with an over-reliance on graphics and sound content effectively bar these people from using them.

Using the World Wide Web

Browsing (or 'surfing') the World Wide Web has become the most popular way of using the Internet. Most people will move from one 'page' (or screen) to another simply through the use of a mouse using a program known as a 'Web browser'. Netscape Navigator and Microsoft Internet Explorer are the two most popular browsers and are fairly similar in appearance. However, some people will browse the Web through specially designed speech synthesizers, their television sets or even mobile telephones. These browsers simply request a document from a computer on the Internet and then display (or speak) it to the user. Whichever way the Web is accessed, the user-friendly nature of its interface is mainly due to one feature: the hyperlink. The author of a Web page can embed the location of another page 'behind' the text they are writing – similar to footnotes or cross-references in a book – but a Web hyperlink is very powerful since it is possible to reference any document on the Web in this way. When the Web was first constructed it was very clear where hyperlinks were on the page (they were sometimes coloured blue and underlined or marked with [square brackets]). Now that commercial interests are beginning to drive Web development, modern design techniques are being employed to make Web pages more attractive. The old-fashioned blue text hyperlink is becoming a thing of the past and it is sometimes necessary to move the mouse across the screen to uncover 'hidden' hyperlinks in order to navigate through the site.

The hyperlink contains the location of the computer which it references on the Internet, together with the position of the document on the computer. These two pieces of information together make up the URL or 'uniform resource locator' of the document. A typical URL might look like: http://www.ioe.ac.uk/ssru.html. The document with such a URL can be retrieved by an Internet protocol, the hypertext transfer protocol, which is indicated by the prefix http. This prefix can be omitted sometimes as some Web browsers will automatically use http. The next three or four sets of letters separated by a full stop together make up the address of the computer on the Internet. 'www.ioe.ac.uk' could be thought of as meaning 'the Web server . Institute of Education . an academic site . in the United Kingdom'. Most countries will have a two letter code (for example, fr for France, de for Germany) in this part of the URL and it is a useful indicator of where in the world the Web page is coming from. The exception to this is the USA, which pioneered some of the early development of the Internet. In the same way that Britain – which pioneered a postal system with the penny black stamp – is the one country whose stamps do not indicate their origin, Web addresses in the USA tend not to use the .us suffix. For example, the Web server at the Massachusetts Institute of Technology is identified as 'web.mit.edu' (academic sites in the USA are denoted by .edu rather than .ac). The other common suffix is .com: a commercial site.

The last part of the URL is the location of the document on the computer. This part can be very long and is made up of meaningful words or a jumble of letters, numbers and symbols, interpretable only by a computer.

Getting online

There are a number of ways of accessing the Internet, or 'getting on-line' as it is commonly described. Most people at the moment will use a computer which is connected to a modem plugged into a normal telephone socket. The modem translates the digital signal from the computer into sound, which is then transmitted down the telephone wire and on to the Internet. It also receives signals from the Internet and translates them into a format which the computer can understand. At the other end of the telephone wire is another modem belonging to an *internet service provider*, or ISP for short. This company has a permanent link to the Internet and it allows customers to use this link. At the time of writing most companies offer apparently free access to the Internet, making a profit out of the cost of the phone call to connect to their modems. This seems likely to change, with a number of companies offering freephone Internet access and recouping their costs through other means, such as advertising.

The UK government has recently stated that it wishes to see all households connected to the Internet by 2004 with 'broadband' connections. A broadband connection is very different to a connection over a telephone wire with a normal modem. These connections tend to be 'always on' – i.e. the connection is 24 hours a day – and are also much faster than a connection with a standard modem, so Web pages do not take as long to download. Currently it is possible to buy a broadband Internet connection from BT and cable companies in some areas, but it is expensive: typically £150–200 to buy the equipment and £30–40 per month for access. It should be noted though that there are no call charges on top of this – a computer can be connected to the Internet 24 hours a day using this method for the same cost as if it were only connected for a few minutes. In addition to the above, it is possible to access the Internet through certain digital cable TV services, satellite dishes and even in a very limited way on mobile phones.

Locating evidence on the Internet

Please also refer to our website (http://eppi.ioe.ac.uk/) for more information on this subject.

Most websites will have a *home page* which describes the content of the site, how to move (navigate) around the site and often how to search for information which the site contains. An *ISP* will usually have a home page, which will be the first screen a new user sees when using their service, so this is often the first contact a new user will have when using the Internet. It is often possible to access most of the Web simply by following hyperlinks found on the home pages of an ISP. However, since there are so many websites to look at, using the Internet in this way would be like following shelves in a library and looking at what happens to come to view by looking at the covers of books.

Fortunately, there a number of websites, known as *search engines*, which are devoted to storing information about other sites. Using a search engine could be compared with using a library catalogue – with the proviso that the catalogue is not fully comprehensive and is going out of date by the second. A number of search engines exist but none can cover all Internet sites and all use slightly different ways of classifying and displaying their content. This presents some of the same problems that were identified in Chapter 4: there is a tension between ensuring that the scope of a search is wide enough to capture the information in question, while at the same time not being so inclusive that it yields unmanageable numbers of results. In addition to problems of quantity there are inevitable issues of quality – of ensuring that the information is accurate, relevant and up-to-date.

The major commercial search engines are valuable first ports of call for general information. Yahoo and Lycos are two of the largest and use slightly different ways of structuring their information. Yahoo is a directory-based system where information is entered in a structured way by people who make a decision regarding the classification of each site. Lycos, on the other hand, is the product of a mainly automated system using a computer program (a 'crawler') which visits as many pages on the Internet as it can find and indexes the results as it goes. The search results that are obtained from the two engines reflect the different ways in which they are maintained. Searches are more likely to be specific and accurate on Yahoo because each site has been carefully categorized. However, Yahoo needs website administrators to inform the system of a new site, as otherwise it will not appear in their lists. (Yahoo also contains the results of automatic searching, but not in a categorized form.) The results of searching Lycos are more likely to be comprehensive as Lycos does not depend on human communication, but they can be very imprecise as the coding on Lycos is dependent on computer indexes of the text in a page. (Note that these systems are constantly becoming more sophisticated. For example, it is now possible to inform the Lycos crawler of the address of a home page, and it will visit and index any other pages in the site automatically.)

Yahoo can be found at http://www.yahoo.co.uk/ and is a useful starting place for a search on the Internet. Like many search engines, its home page contains a box in which search terms can be entered and a list of categories through which it is possible to browse. Entering 'healthy eating' as a search term will yield about 110,000 websites listed in no particular order, 20 at a time. Conducting the same search on Lycos (http://www.lycos.co.uk/) yields 4,155 sites – quite a difference, even though the search on Yahoo included Ireland in addition to the UK. Though 110,000 websites is an impossibly large number to look through, the Yahoo system of manually categorizing entries paid off in that it singled out the Health Development Agency's 'LifeBytes' website[6] from the 110,000 other sites as being particularly relevant to the search. These searches were carried out on 31 August 2000 at 18:00 BST and are a good illustration of how quickly the Internet changes. By 27 September the same search on Yahoo yielded only about 33,300 websites, but it had added another four to its categorized section on healthy eating. Clearly Yahoo has changed either its catalogue or the way in which searches operate.

Sooner or later, most people will come across a link to a page which cannot be displayed after clicking on the link. These are known as broken links and an error is usually shown. Sometimes this is because the page has been deleted and moved to another site, and sometimes simply because the page has been moved somewhere else on the server. For example, an article on the website of the *British Medical Journal*[7] (*BMJ*) refers to Health A to Z on the Web as http://www.healthatoz.com/aboutus.htm. Unfortunately, Health A to Z has renamed or changed the 'aboutus.htm' page and clicking on the link from the *BMJ* website in August 2000 simply returned an error ('404 Not Found. The Web server cannot find the file or script you asked for. Please check the URL to ensure that the path is correct'). In circumstances like this it is a good idea to take advantage of the 'default' home page feature which is built in to most Web servers (and Web browsers). If no reference to a specific page is given (in this case 'aboutus.htm') the Web server will return the home page for that area of the site. In this example, simply entering http://www.healthatoz.com/ – the Internet address for the Health A to Z server rather than any specific page – will give us the home page of Health A to Z and it is possible to navigate through to the 'aboutus.htm' page from there (it had changed to http://www.healthatoz.com/atoz/aboutus.asp).

Yahoo and Lycos and other search engines are also described as 'gateways' to the Internet: they present ways through which the Internet can be accessed and provide some structure to the unstructured mass of information found there. There are also health-specific gateways, which have usually been compiled by people working in the health field. These sites are a lot smaller than the large commercial sites, but even though they have a specific focus and have been manually rather than automatically compiled, they cannot be relied upon to be any more comprehensive than the large search engines. The lists of links to sites which they hold are limited by the interest and knowledge of the people who have compiled them. It is not always clear why some sites have been included and others omitted, so at the moment Internet users need to keep their own records of particularly useful sites or gateways. Fortunately, the popular Web browsers have a built-in function to store the location of useful sites: *bookmarks* (Netscape) or *favorites* (Internet Explorer). This facility allows a Web browser to remember a website and useful gateways which can then be located quickly when carrying out a search. It is usually best to store the home page of a website as a bookmark rather than a specific page buried deep within a site since pages are often moved around, leading to 'Not Found' errors (see above) when the bookmark is used. There are now so many gateways on the Web that some sites are being set up as gateways to gateways, an example of which is Pinakes.[8] Rather than using a large number of gateways quickly, though, it is usually best to identify the best ones for a particular subject area and use them thoroughly.

As with all websites, the quality of health-specific gateways can be variable. Some are an unordered list of 'useful links' which provide little or no information about the listed sites: for example, why the sites are on the list and what kind of information they contain. In contrast to this, the 'Netting the Evidence' website maintained by Andrew Booth at the University of Sheffield[9] has grown from being the aforementioned list of links into a site which structures, categorizes (searching, appraising, implementing etc.) and describes the websites it lists, alongside a 'library' of links to articles on critical appraisal and other aspects of evidence-based practice. A list of *mirror* sites (places in other parts of the world where a copy of a site can be found) shows that this site is recognized internationally as being an exceptionally valuable resource in its field.

Though the Sheffield website is a valuable resource, its maintainers would not claim that it contains links to every site that health researchers and practitioners would need to visit. Indeed, some health promotion material is merely part of more general medical sites and it is necessary to hunt carefully to find relevant information. There are few health promotion specific gateways for the same reason. This lack of a central place to find information is a problem that has been recognized by a number of people – often resulting in yet more gateways to be added to bookmark lists. The proposed website of the new Health Development Agency, 'Evidence Base', aims to be the comprehensive site which is needed, but as this site is still under construction at the time of writing it is impossible to say whether it will meet this aim, or will simply become one of a growing list of sites to consult when a search is being undertaken. This site also plans to indicate the quality of the sites to which it links. In many ways this is more problematic than having a comprehensive database of links – as can be seen by a number of attempts to classify quality in other parts of the world.

In addition to displaying static pages of text held on computers around the world, the Internet is becoming a place where it is possible to meet people working in the same field and exchange views and information. There are numerous ways to interact with people over the Internet, ranging from email lists, video conferencing and chat rooms (where it is possible to have a 'live' conversation with several people) to 'newsgroups' (open forum discussions which look a little like email). Whichever medium is used, a written and unwritten code of conduct has developed regarding acceptable ways to interact with other people over the Internet: this is known as *netiquette*. For example, it is a good idea for a *newbie* (a novice user) to read the *FAQ* (frequently asked questions) for a newsgroup or email list before writing a question, since the question may have already been asked and answered many times before. Detailed descriptions of acceptable behaviour may be found by entering the term 'netiquette' on one of the search engines mentioned earlier in this chapter.

The development of 'on-line communities' has been one of the most interesting features of the Internet as it has grown over the past decade. Prior to this, the mutual exchange of support and views had been confined mainly to academics and those most knowledgeable about the technologies involved. The NetDoctor site[10] is a good example of how this is changing. It contains a number of features which go beyond the static perusal of Web pages: a facility to send emails of health news to those subscribed to a list and a part of the website where it is possible to 'ask the doctor' are two examples of this. The most interactive areas are the chat sessions and discussion forums. For example, on the day this paragraph was written two doctors were holding a live chat session on migraine to which it was possible to submit questions by email. There are also 26 open discussion forums around which a community of peers is forming, offering advice and support covering many aspects of health. Another type of online community is centred on email lists. These are groups of people who correspond with each other by email in such a way that the whole group receives each email. Chains of correspondence build up in which all the group are able to participate. Mailbase[11] is a good first port of call when looking for an email list, though there are many linked to individual websites. It is worth checking how busy a mailing list is before joining. Sometimes the number of messages can run into hundreds per day!

Questionable quality and questionable ethics

In a survey in 1997, Piero Impicciator and colleagues sought to examine the reliability of health care advice on the World Wide Web and assess its possible benefits. They compared the advice being given on 41 Web pages they uncovered (with searches on Yahoo and Excite) with that contained in published guidelines for managing fever in children at home. They found that only four pages provided 'complete and accurate information' and suggested that there was an 'urgent need to check public oriented healthcare information on the Internet for accuracy, completeness, and consistency.'[12]

The issue of whether or not information found on the Internet should be controlled never seems to be far from the news. This growing concern can be observed by looking through the online archive at the *BMJ*'s website. When the Internet was relatively new the articles concentrated on how to use this new medium of communication. In the past few years there have been more articles expressing concern at some of the information which has become available. For instance, Roger Dobson wrote[13] to express his concern that the Internet might be encouraging suicide. While his citation of the website of the Church of Euthanasia in the article may be a little misleading,[14] he is almost certainly correct in his assertion that there are thousands of sites which will detail suicide techniques in some form or other. (This topic also highlights the issue of liability for publication on the Internet: Imperial College, London houses a large archive of mirror sites around the world and one document[15] is possibly illegal in England and other countries due to laws regarding assisting suicide.) Even though there is evidence that talking to young people about suicide can encourage it (Harden *et al.* 2000),[16] it does not necessarily follow that Internet sites dealing with the subject should be banned. As has been mentioned elsewhere in this book, even well intentioned interventions can be harmful and have unforeseen consequences.

A search on the website of the *BMJ* reveals many calls for quality assessment of the advice being given on unregulated websites. Indeed, a number of organizations are working to do this. The Internet Healthcare Coalition[17] is seeking to promote self-regulation in this area in an attempt to preempt legislation. The UK-based 'DISCERN on the Internet Project'[18] is taking a different approach by seeking to give consumers a tool with which they can assess critically the information they find on the Internet. The World Health Organization offers criteria[19] which are similar to DISCERN in that they have been adapted from criteria developed for use with printed material. Many of the issues of accuracy, reliability, relevance, clarity and bias are the same for both media. Chapter 6 contains a detailed discussion of critical appraisal which is applicable to information found on the Internet as well as in printed form.

Jadad and Gagliardi (1998) conclude that 'Many incompletely developed instruments to evaluate health information exist on the Internet. It is unclear, however, whether they should exist in the first place, whether they measure what they claim to measure, or whether they lead to more good than harm.' A year later Paul Ki and colleagues[20] conducted a similar review of published criteria for evaluating health-related websites, but came to more positive conclusions. While the existence of the 29 rating tools which they found might appear to be a source of confusion in itself, they found that 132 of the 165 criteria extracted could be grouped into one of 12 specific categories. Most common were those criteria dealing with the 'content, design and aesthetics' of a website, followed by 'disclosure of authors, sponsors or developers'. This last category is important because it is very easy to conceal the source of information and funding on a website. For example, at the time of writing, the Medezone[21] site states that the site will be funded in the future by income from job advertisements, but makes no mention of who is funding it at the moment. All websites will reflect the biases and commercial interests of those who support them. This is important information for users to have when evaluating what a particular page is telling them, and the deliberate or accidental concealment of these details makes it impossible for users to judge the value of a site properly. Indeed, they may take the information contained within a site at face value, unaware of the commercial or value-driven judgements which underlie its inclusion, and why other information may have been excluded. It is possible that tobacco companies will make their research available on the Internet in the future.[22] This is a very clear example of why it is important to bear in mind the source of information and how this might affect its validity. Here it is clear that there is at least the possibility of a conflict of interests – in other cases it may not be so obvious. A case in point is the DrKoop story, detailed in several places on the *BMJ* website.[23] It was very difficult to detect that certain articles on the DrKoop website were in effect advertisements for hospitals that had paid large sums of money to be included in this way.

Many websites now require users to register themselves, usually asking for at least a name and an email address for verification. The intricacies of security on the Internet are beyond the scope of this chapter, but a useful tip is always to read the privacy policy, which should be available alongside any requests for identifying information. It is also worth recording the usernames and passwords that are often picked quickly in order to access a site. To keep personal email and other accounts secure, never use the same details for registration purposes in other places. Before long most users of the Internet will encounter *SPAM* (unsolicited) emails. Sites with a lax privacy policy will often sell registered email addresses to marketing firms.

The question of why some services are offered on certain websites is also important. Many websites will offer a number of features, such as WWW, Medline and library searches and email updates of news. These features are freely available elsewhere on the Web (in fact the search started on one site will often be conducted on another), and the reason a site offers links to these services is simply to encourage people to return. It may be that the proliferation of links to the free version of Medline may not be very helpful. As has been noted elsewhere, the results of one or two primary studies found in a Medline search may not be the most reliable indication of 'what works'. Of more value might be a review found, for example, on the Cochrane Library,[24] DARE[25] or the Register of Reviews of Effectiveness at the EPPI-Centre.[26]

Even when the information contained in a website is correct, problems still may arise due to the fact that information which is accurate in one country does not apply in another. For example, some drugs are commonly available in America while they are restricted or not yet approved in the UK.

Some concern is expressed by doctors in the on-line *BMJ* that patients are attending surgery armed with information taken from the Internet. Some are alarmed that as information on best practice becomes more accessible through the Internet there is an increased chance of medical practitioners being challenged in court: 'While patients may be motivated to seek out the most recent literature for their condition and can invest considerable effort in that search, most practising doctors cannot.' This is a problem not only because patients may access the information rather than doctors, but doctors may find it difficult to respond when they have not had time to appraise the information, and they feel undermined in a difficult situation – ironically, in this era of increased information, communication sometimes suffers.

Mention should also be made of the difficulties inherent in quoting URLs as sources for further information. The dynamic nature of the Web means that a link could be broken at any time – possibly irrecoverably. Indeed, it is possible that some of the links contained within this book will be out-of-date by the time of publication. The stating of search strategies on Internet sites is not a reliable way of describing what has been done because of the way that databases change – sometimes on a daily basis. These are issues that stem from the newness of the medium: many websites are in a constant state of flux as administrators and designers learn better ways of organizing and presenting their information. Generating a system for ensuring the replicability of search strategies is even more problematic, as any system must make it possible for a search to be repeated: something which is impossible at the moment due to the way in which most databases are constructed.

Though the previous paragraphs highlight a number of important problems facing the Internet at the moment, there are many examples of the Internet saving lives and improving the quality and accessibility of information for people all over the world. A brief examination of how the Internet has aided the Cochrane Collaboration demonstrates this. Communication across the Collaboration has been greatly enhanced by the contribution that email and the Web have made, and smaller working groups have their own discussion lists which enable debate to occur without the need for face-to-face meetings. The software used to write a systematic review in the Cochrane format is downloadable, and in the UK health care professionals have free access to the Cochrane Library over the Internet. While global collaboration was possible before the advent of the Internet, it has made the process much faster and more efficient, enabling the Collaboration to grow much faster and produce more reviews in a shorter time than would otherwise have been possible.

The Internet (together with the development of sophisticated computerized searching techniques) has also revolutionized the way in which research is conducted, enabling far more detailed examinations of available literature to be carried out, and many more immediate and global contacts to be made. More interactivity can be expected in the future as more people gain access and the speed of that access increases. This can be seen already in some cases where trials are being conducted using the Web as the primary medium for consultation and advice. Though many issues must be borne in mind when using it, the Internet can be a valuable resource – and the possibilities for its use have only just begun to be explored.

Notes

1   http://www.isoc.org/zakon/Internet/History/HIT.html
2   http://www.nua.ie/surveys/
3   http://www.mcconnellinternational.com/ereadiness/EReadinessReport.htm
4   http://news.bbc.co.uk/hi/english/sci/tech/newsid_760000/760867.stm
5   http://virtualsociety.sbs.ox.ac.uk/research/virtsoc/
6   http://www.lifebytes.gov.uk/
7   http://www.bmj.com/cgi/content/full/318/7184/647/DC1/1
8   http://www.hw.ac.uk/libWWW/irn/pinakes/pinakes.html
9   http://www.shef.ac.uk/~scharr/ir/netting/
10 http://www.netdoctor.co.uk/
11 http://www.mailbase.ac.uk/ and http://www.jismail.ac.uk/default.htm
12 http://www.bmj.com/cgi/content/full/314/7098/1875
13 BMJ 1999;319:337, http://www.bmj.com/cgi/content/full/319/7206/337
14 http://www.churchofeuthanasia.org/
15 http://sunsite.doc.ic.ac.uk/usenet/news-faqs/alt.suicide.holiday/Encouraging_
    Suicide_—_Frequently_Asked_Questions (not found 30 March 2001)
16 Available on-line at http://eppi.ioe.ac.uk/
17 http://www.ihealthcoalition.org/
18 http://www.discern.org.uk/
19 http://www.who.int/hlt/virtuallibrary/English/evalulat.htm
20 http://www.bmj.com/cgi/content/full/318/7184/647
21 http://www.medezone.com/
22 http://www.bmj.com/cgi/content/full/320/7231/336/f
23 http://www.bmj.com/cgi/content/short/319/7212/727
24 The Cochrane Library is not freely available on the Internet at the time of writing.
    Please see http://www.update-software.com/cochrane/cochrane-frame.html for
    more details.
25 http://agatha.york.ac.uk/darehp.htm
26 http://eppi.ioe.ac.uk/

References

Harden, A., Weston, R. and Oakley, A. (1999) *A Review of the Effectiveness and Appropriateness of Peer-delivered Health Promotion Interventions for Young People*. London: EPI-Centre, Social Science Research Unit.

Jadad, A. R. and Gagliardi, A. (1998) Rating health information on the Internet: navigating to knowledge or to Babel? *Journal of the American Medical Association*, 279(8), 611–14.

▶ 6

▷ Critical appraisal of research evidence: finding useful and reliable answers

▷ Sandy Oliver and Greet Peersman

As discussed in Chapter 3, there is a range of different types of information that can be used to make decisions about ways of improving people's health and reducing disease and disability. When you turn to the research literature for help in tackling an individual or local problem, knowing where and how to look for answers requires being clear about the type of information sought (see Chapter 4). Once the relevant research papers are obtained, the next step is to judge whether we can trust the results, what they mean and whether they are applicable in the given circumstances, and hence can be used for explaining and justifying subsequent decisions. This is an important process as the quality of research varies. As Tricia Greenhalgh (1997: 34) puts it:

> bad science is bad science regardless of whether the study examined an important clinical issue, whether the results are statistically significant, whether things changed in the direction you would have liked them to, and whether, if true, the findings promise immeasurable benefits for patients or savings for the health service.

Acting on unreliable evidence at best distorts professional values and practices, and at worst can actually cause harm to those receiving care (CASP 1999).

Weighing up (critically appraising) evidence in order to assess its closeness to the truth (validity) and its usefulness (applicability) in the given circumstances is a process that is not unique to reading research papers. Indeed, people approach just about any type of reading with this frame of mind, even if mostly subconsciously. What makes 'critical appraisal' of research papers a more formal process is the use of a structured, systematic approach, typically including detailed questions to help to make a judgement on three levels of inquiry: (a) are the results sound; (b) what are the results; and (c) will the results help me (CASP 1999)? Critical appraisal in this context started with clinicians checking the research evidence underpinning drug treatments. Since then the framework of critical appraisal has been applied in varying degrees to other health care procedures and ways of organizing services, including, but to a lesser extent, qualitative research on people's values, beliefs and motivations.

Critical appraisal is not about fault finding; nor should it result in destructive nihilism, concluding that there isn't anything to be learned from 'imperfect' research. Greenhalgh (1997: 35) writes 'It is much easier to pick holes in other people's work than to do a methodologically perfect piece of research oneself'. She continues:

> When I teach critical appraisal there is usually someone in the group who finds it profoundly discourteous to criticise research projects into which dedicated scientists have put the best years of their lives. On a more pragmatic note, there may be good practical reasons why the authors of the study have 'cut corners' and they know as well as you do that their work would have been more scientifically valid if they hadn't.

It is important to bear in mind the purpose of critical appraisal, which is to help us to make important judgements and be explicit and precise about the evidence on which decisions are based. By addressing research reports systematically, we can be sure of not only reading what is presented, but also noticing what other useful information is missing.

This chapter demonstrates the critical appraisal of different types of research (experimental, observational, qualitative) using prevention of hip fractures in older people as an example. It presents a set of questions that may be asked of each type of research report for checking the validity of the results, their meaning and their relevance to specific queries.

Recognizing the questions before looking for the answers

Osteoporosis and associated fractures are a major cause of death, illness and disability, and a cause of huge medical expense worldwide. Bone fractures are the main complication, and given that they are most common in older people, it is predicted that the influence of increasing life expectancy on the number of fractures will be dramatic. For example, the World Health Organization estimates that the number of hip fractures could rise from 1.7 million 1990 to around 6.3 million by 2050 (WHO 1998). In addition to the public health concern, hip fractures also create serious personal problems for many older people, giving them a lot of pain and taking away their physical health, mobility and independence. Given the extent and nature of the problem, 'we' need to 'do something' about hip fractures. What we try to do depends on our skills and opportunities, and what we know about what might help. Pertinent questions are: 'How can we prevent people from falling?'; 'How can we reduce the negative impact of a fall?'; 'What is the best way of treating people who have sustained a hip fracture?' For example, surgeons may want to know about the latest operative procedures, how to do them and how their success compares with more traditional techniques. Nursing home staff may ask whether hip-protecting padding prevents fractures during falls. Older people themselves may have their own views about keeping themselves safe and how they can continue to act as independent adults and make their own choices. Issues of comfort and ease of using protective devices, for example, may be important considerations in their choice of and compliance with such preventive measures. Thus, responsible decisions about how to intervene in people's lives benefit from a sound understanding of the problem from the perspectives of all those involved, whether they are developing, delivering, evaluating or potentially receiving the intervention. The ideologies held by all those involved must be respected, and steer the information generated through research about the feasibility, acceptability and effectiveness of available interventions.

Does it work? Appraising a trial

To answer, for example, the question 'do hip protectors prevent fractures?', we could seek research that has asked women who have suffered hip fractures whether they ever used hip protectors. This type of study looks into the past to seek causes for health problems occurring today – this is a retrospective study. It would tell us nothing about women who did not suffer fractures. Even if women who did not sustain fractures were also included in the study, it would be difficult to obtain reliable information about how often, if at all, women wore protectors in the past, what type of protectors, in what circumstances and since when. The conclusions of such a retrospective study about the protective value of hip padding could only be conjecture. Alternatively, we could look for research that compares women who wear hip protectors with others who do not, and follows them over time to see what happens in terms of subsequent falls and injuries – this is a prospective and observational study. There still remains a risk of being misled if women who wear hip protectors tend to be more cautious generally, not only wearing hip protectors but also having additional handrails fitted in their homes, always wearing flat and well fitting shoes, never carrying more than one item at a time or taking the stairs a little slower, and thereby suffer fewer fractures for all manner of reasons. To avoid such problems we should look for experimental studies such as controlled trials in which people are 'allocated' to wearing hip protectors or not, and then followed up over time. But before we attribute cause and effect, a number of questions need to be asked of the 'test' or evaluation report. Figure 6.1

Figure 6.1   Questions for appraising an intervention test report

Are the results of the outcome evaluation valid?
I   Did the evaluation address a clearly focused issue?
2   Were the people receiving the intervention compared with an equivalent control or comparison group?
3   Were all the people who entered the evaluation properly accounted for and attributed at its conclusion?
4   Was the intervention described clearly?
5   Is it clear how the control group and experimental groups did or did not change after the intervention?

What are the results?
6   How large was the impact of the intervention?
7   How precise are the results?

Will the results help me?
8   Can the results be applied to the local population?
9   Were all important outcomes considered?
10 Are the benefits worth the harms and costs?

lists brief questions to help readers to judge how confident they are in the scientific rigour and the value of the test results. The questions are derived from methodological research about testing the effects of interventions, and have been refined over years of use by clinicians (Guyatt *et al.* 1993; Oxman *et al.* 1994), purchasers of health care (Milne *et al.* 1995), health promotion professionals (Oliver *et al.* 1996) and service users (Milne and Oliver 1996). The remainder of this section applies these questions to a practical example of a study by Lauritzen *et al.* (1993), in which the ability of hip protectors to prevent fractures was assessed in residents of a nursing home in Copenhagen, Denmark.

Did the evaluation address a clearly focused issue?

In other words, is the report clear about whose health is being tested (the population), how they were 'helped' (the interventions) and how their health was subsequently assessed (the outcomes)? These basics are essential for describing what is having an effect on whom and, if at all, how much. In this case, the population was residents of a nursing home in Copenhagen, between the ages of 50 and 99 years, and twice as many women as men. The intervention was padding worn around the hip to reduce the impact of a fall and thereby the chance of fracturing the hip. The outcomes recorded were the number of hip and other fractures incurred during a period of eleven months and, in a subgroup, the number of falls and repeat falls, the type of impact and the type of trauma. 'Compliance' with wearing the protectors was also assessed.

Were the people receiving the intervention compared with an equivalent control or comparison group?

The groups may be equivalent if the people were selected in similar ways, and their demographic characteristics and health status are very similar. If not, hip protectors may not have been put to a fair test. They may have been given to people who were older than average, who may have been less likely to try walking alone or more likely to fall if they did. In the Copenhagen trial, wards of the nursing home were allocated at random to receive (or not) hip protectors; a ward was selected when its number was drawn by a doctor who was not involved in the study. Because, on average, the groups in a randomized controlled trial (RCT) are identical apart from the intervention, any differences in outcome are, in theory, attributable to the intervention (Greenhalgh 1997). The groups in the trial were unequal in size for economic reasons; only 10 of the 28 wards were randomly chosen to receive hip protectors. However, they had a similar age and sex distribution, which is crucial, as these variables are known to interact with the outcomes under study.

If the report is of a clearly focused controlled trial, as in this case, it is worth reading further and conducting a more detailed check of the findings and their applicability.

Were all the people who entered the evaluation properly accounted for and attributed at its conclusion?

This involves comparing the number of people recruited (participation rate), the number of people allocated to the different groups, the number of people reported in the outcome data tables and the number of people who dropped out (attrition rate), who they were and why. Perhaps more people given hip protectors dropped out of the trial, because they did not want the bother of wearing them. Or perhaps more older people dropped out because they moved to alternative accommodation during the trial. The Copenhagen trial had 247 residents (167 women, 80 men) in the intervention group, and 418 residents (277 women, 141 men) in the control group (i.e. 665 people overall). Hip and other fractures were reported for 665 residents. However, the authors indicated that for any deaths occurring during the study period of 11 months, available places in the nursing home were immediately filled by new arrivals from a waiting list and included in the study. This means that some people may not have been followed up for the entire study period. The authors did not mention how many such cases occurred.

In addition to the 'main study', a subgroup of 116 residents (45 intervention participants, 71 participants in the control group) was followed up for fall-related data.

Was the intervention described clearly?

For reports of health promotion evaluations to be useful elsewhere, it is particularly important that they describe the intervention clearly. Commercially available hip protectors may be easy to obtain for subsequent use by others, but more complex care, such as exercise regimes, needs more detail if readers are to replicate it elsewhere. For this trial, the hip protectors had an outer shield of polypropylene and an inner part of plastozote, and were fixed in special underwear. Every resident in the intervention group was given three sets of underpants and one pair of hip protectors. The external hip protector was designed to divert direct impact away from the hip bone during a fall by transmitting released energy to the soft tissue and muscles.

Is it clear how the control and experimental groups did or did not change after the intervention?

Detecting an intervention effect requires observing a difference in subsequent health (in this case, number of fractures) between equivalent intervention and control/comparison groups, or observing differences in behaviour (in this case, frequency of falls). Some measures are usefully made before and after an intervention (e.g. frequency of falls) but for others (such as fractures) prior measurement does not make sense.

How large was the impact of the intervention?

When it is clear that a controlled trial has been well conducted, it is worth asking how large the difference, if any, was for each of the outcomes measured? In this example, eight (3 per cent) residents in the intervention group had a hip fracture (none was wearing hip protectors at the time) and 31 (7 per cent) in the control group; the corresponding data for non-hip fractures were 15 (6 per cent) and 27 (6 per cent), respectively. The authors also presented the relative risk (RR) of hip fractures in the intervention group. If intervening had no measurable effect, the odds of hip fractures in the intervention group and the control group would be identical, i.e. one. Here, the RR was 0.46 for women (i.e. 54 per cent of hip fractures averted), 0.29 for men (71 per cent of hip fractures averted) and 0.44 overall (56 per cent of hip fractures averted), indicating that the hip protectors did indeed have a protective effect.

   In terms of falls, recorded in the subgroup, 64 falls occurred in the intervention group and 90 in the control group; repeat falls made up 35 per cent of falls in the intervention group and 46 per cent in the control group. Six hip fractures were associated with impact to the hip; only one occurred in a resident in the intervention group. No fractures occurred in the instances when a protector was being worn.

How precise are the results?

In other words, how sure are we of the results? This question is related to the size of the confidence interval. Usually, research studies indicate the size of the 99 per cent or the 95 per cent confidence interval (CI). The 95 per cent CI, for example, means that if the trial were repeated 100 times we would expect the result to fall within this range 95 times. In this trial, 95 times out of 100 we would expect the RR for hip fractures in both men and women in the intervention group as compared to the control group to fall between 0.01 and 0.94. This is a very broad range, so the results of this study are not very precise. As a matter of fact, the 95 per cent CIs for the RR in women and men separately (0.20–1.00 and 0.04–2.5, respectively) include one (the point at which the intervention has no effect), so we cannot conclude with confidence that the intervention had beneficial effects. Caution in the interpretation of the results is therefore warranted. The authors do, however, indicate that none of the residents sustaining hip fractures was actually wearing the hip protector at the time, which sheds a different light on these findings.

Can the results be applied to the local population?

Even if positive results are found, they can only be promising if they are relevant to the circumstances of whoever is appraising the report. Can the results be applied to the local population? Are the people involved in the evaluation similar enough to others at risk? At the time of this trial, the relative risk of hip fractures in the nursing home was about three times that of the local general population. Thus the results of this trial seem to apply only to those at vastly increased risk of hip fracture.

Were all important outcomes considered?

If not, should this affect a decision about offering hip protectors? At first glance hip protectors seem to benefit people at risk of falling, but a note in the paper about 'compliance' suggests there may be disadvantages too. Only 45 of the 247 people given hip protectors were monitored throughout the study, and only 11 (24 per cent) of these wore them regularly. What were the problems? Were they uncomfortable or difficult to use, or did they have undesirable side-effects? In a trial that only seeks to measure the desirable outcomes, we can only guess the possible harms. The authors noted that nurses were more keen to make recurrent fallers wear hip protectors, and that the process of putting on the hip protectors may have been too difficult for some people to do.

Are the benefits worth the harms and costs?

Ultimately, the benefits need to be balanced with the harms and the costs. Even if side-effects have been measured, such a value judgement is unlikely to be addressed by the evaluation, and it calls for some speculation. Appraising this trial raises more questions: are hip protectors acceptable to old people or do they bring unseen problems and harms; and is this trial an isolated example or have others investigated the same intervention, and come to the same conclusions, or not?

What else might work? Appraising a review

Rather than relying on the findings of a single study, a more cautious approach recommends considering all similar studies. A short-cut to their findings is a literature review, where the work of drawing together the relevant literature has already been done. Six years after the Copenhagen study was published, a review of the effects of hip protectors which meets high standards for its systematic approach was published in *The Cochrane Library* (Parker *et al.* 2000). This review confirmed that hip padding does protect hips from fracture but noted that older people commonly choose not to use them: some pads were uncomfortable or badly fitting, or made dressing difficult for patients who were mainly bedridden, confused or infirm. They could be intolerable when hot, and could cause skin irritation. A common-sense response to this is to question why all that money was spent on research when asking people what they felt about hip protectors at the beginning might have resulted in the development and trialling of more appropriate equipment. Such difficulties call for more qualitative research and the subsequent development of more acceptable protective measures, before they are tested to see if they are equally effective in preventing hip fractures. They also call for other types of interventions to prevent falls and hip fractures.

   Literature reviews in the area of prevention of falls and fractures in older people have taken a variety of approaches. Above we saw how a review of the literature addressed the effects of hip padding on hip fractures (Parker *et al.* 2000); other specific questions include asking about the effects of nutritional supplements (Avenell and Handoll 2000), hormone replacement therapy (Tugwell *et al.* 2000), vitamin D (Gillespie *et al.* 2000b) or exercise (Tai *et al.* 2000). An alternative, broader approach is defining the population of interest (older people) and the outcomes of interest (accidents, falls or injuries) and seeking any interventions that have been tested with this population for an impact on these outcomes (Gillespie *et al.* 2000a). If other ways are found for reducing hip fractures, guidance may be sought about the practical implications: who should deliver an intervention; with

Figure 6.2   Questions for appraising a literature review

Are the results of the review valid?
1 Did the review address a clearly focused issue?
2 Did the authors select the right sort of studies for the review?
3 Do you think the important, relevant studies were included?
4 Did the review's authors do enough to assess the quality of the included studies?
5 Were the results similar from study to study?

What are the results?
6 What is the overall result of the review?
7 How precise are the results?

Will the results help locally?
8 Can the results be applied to the local population?
9 Were all important outcomes considered?
10 Are the benefits worth the harms and costs?

what resources and training; and how many people might they be expected to reach? The health promotion literature has many such studies, published and unpublished, investigating the processes involved, and they provide invaluable guidance for people setting up new initiatives.

As with using the findings of a primary study in planning services, it is important not to be misled by biases in a literature review. If a few studies that are easily found are simply summarized, there is the risk of drawing conclusions from a few weak studies and missing others altogether; perhaps some of these may contradict the ones we found. Reviews that are conducted well meet criteria for good searching and quality checks of the studies they consider; and these reviews can be distinguished from unreliable reviews by appropriate critical appraisal. A little scepticism, and checking the reliability of the review step-by-step, similar to appraising primary studies, is necessary to distinguish comprehensive, soundly conducted reviews from thoughtful essays or flawed pieces of research. An example of questions for critically appraising a review is given in Figure 6.2. These questions address important steps in conducting a review, which are explained in detail in Chapter 7.

What do people want? Appraising a qualitative study

The critical appraisal described so far applies to reports of interventions whose parameters (processes and outcomes) have been determined in advance. The prior question is what parameters should we be considering? Decisions about how to intervene in people's lives ethically require the views of these people themselves, and it is necessary for them to have a role in the decision-making. This may be by involving them directly in the development and evaluation of an intervention (see Chapter 10), or indirectly by applying the findings of qualitative research which seeks to understand people's values and preferences. Some research sets out to discover issues of concern to the different people involved in coping with a problem. It aims to achieve a sound understanding of the problem and issues of importance.

For instance, Hey (1994b) adopted a qualitative methodology when wishing to explore the choices older people have for their care in the community. A prior literature review had revealed that little is known about how older people are involved in decisions about their care, if at all (Hey 1994a). She set out to discover how the implementation of 'care in the community' was affecting the care of older people in the community. This was a tangible problem which needed to be better defined before any way forward could be proposed. Thus her specific objectives were: to explore the views and experiences of frail older people and those caring for them when making choices about their care; to look at the relationships between mental competence and physical dependence, health, social support and the social circumstances of frail older people; and to make practical and policy recommendations about the involvement of frail older people in choices about their living circumstances. Whether she did it appropriately and in the best way, and whether this was apparent in her report, is difficult to tell. She was well aware of the problems, and a reflective account expanded on some of these (Hey 1999). Her use of the first person assumed 'the impossibility of doing value-free social science investigation', but even this self-awareness did not prepare her for the near impossibility of doing the research at all. The research funders were 'rare in specifically wanting to discover the views of the frail elderly themselves' and their request was thwarted in many ways. Meeting potential research participants depended on the sponsorship of 'gatekeepers', care managers and social workers, who necessarily influenced the sample of people to be interviewed. 'Choice', the issue under investigation, meant little to interviewees who were poor or destitute and did not see themselves as consumers of services. Their plight and their personal histories were so disturbing that Hey found herself distracted from the research task by her compassion. Interpreting interviews demanded she 'listen to the spoken and for the silenced'. How can the quality of such a report be judged?

While advice for doing qualitative research abounds, there is little consensus about how to read qualitative research critically. Criteria have been adopted from both the positivist paradigm and the qualitative paradigm in an attempt to appraise reports of qualitative research, but without reaching a conclusion (Oakley 2000). The question remains: 'how will we know "good" qualitative research when we see it?' (Devers 1999). Two approaches may solve this problem: a structured debate among a broad range of researchers and research users to identify and operationalize criteria for judging the quality of studies (CASP 1999); followed by testing such criteria for their utility in the preparation of systematic reviews (e.g. Harden *et al.* 1999).

What happens in practice? Appraising a service report

Health promotion practitioners need to know more than whether an intervention is effective; they need to know how to replicate it in their local setting. Figure 6.3 suggests questions for systematically considering whether a report offers information about the development and delivery of an intervention – a process intervention. These questions provide a suggested framework only. They have not been validated by rigorous research and they do not appraise the quality of the data collected, but highlight what has been collected, and what has not.

A process evaluation may focus on any aspect of developing and delivering an intervention: the initial planning and consultation; development of materials; education and training; establishing access to the target population; or media and publicity. The planning and consultation may include checking the need for health promotion, seeking the views and knowledge of the target group and identifying what resources are needed and available

Figure 6.3   Questions for appraising a process evaluation

Are the results of the process evaluation reliable?

1 Does the study focus on a health promotion intervention?
2 Does the intervention have clearly stated aims?
3 Does the study describe the key processes involved in *delivering* this intervention?
4 Does the study tell you enough about planning and consultation?
5 Does the study tell you enough about the collaborative effort required for the intervention?
6 Does the study tell you enough about the materials used in the intervention?
7 Does the study tell you enough about how the target population was identified and recruited?
8 Does the study tell you enough about education and training?

What are the results?

9 Were all the processes described and adequately monitored?
10 Was the intervention acceptable?

Will the results help me?

11 Can the results be applied to the local population?
12 Were all important processes considered?
13 If you wanted to know whether this intervention promotes health what outcomes would you want to measure?

---

to deliver the intervention. Some studies describe the collaborative effort required for an intervention: which individuals and/or groups were working together to deliver an intervention (such as multidisciplinary teams) or to enable people to take responsibility for their own health (such as in community developments).

Considerable effort may be made to develop audio, visual and printed material, and some studies describe these and report how they were developed and disseminated. Reaching the intended target population may not be straightforward. Details of how they were reached, introduced to the study and invited to consent to participation would also be useful.

If the success of an intervention may depend on the experience, education and training of those leading the intervention, delivering the intervention or receiving the intervention, this information should be available. Practicalities of recruitment and training for delivering the intervention and reaching the target population may be monitored as part of a process evaluation (see Chapter 10). Success will also depend on how acceptable the intervention was to those responsible for its delivery, and those receiving it.

If all the necessary information is available, it may be possible to replicate the intervention successfully to the benefit of people who are sufficiently similar to those in the original study. A standard set of questions such as those in Figure 6.3 helps to appraise reports in terms of the 'catchall' question 'were all important processes considered?' Without such a framework the gaps would not be apparent.

Conclusions

Using health promotion in older people as an example, this chapter has illustrated the use of some practical tools for assessing the validity and usefulness of different types of research studies which bring together different perspectives in addressing health problems. Key messages include:

- We need to decide which type of research report(s) to seek out to answer specific health questions
- Critical appraisal helps us to bring our judgement to a research report in a structured way: are the results of the research valid; what are the results; will the results help me?

References

Avenell, A. and Handoll, H. (2000) Nutritional supplementation for hip fracture aftercare in the elderly. In *The Cochrane Library*, Issue 1. Oxford: Update Software.

CASP (1999) Evidence-based health care: an open learning resource for health care practitioners. Critical Appraisal Skills Programme and Health Care Libraries Unit. NHS Executive Anglia and Oxford.

Devers, K. (1999) How will we know 'good' qualitative research when we see it? Beginning the dialogue in health services research. *Health Services Research*, 34(5), 1153–88.

Gillespie, L., Gillespie, W., Cumming, R., Lamb, S. and Rowe, B. (2000a) Interventions for preventing falls in the elderly. In *The Cochrane Library*, Issue 1. Oxford: Update Software.

Gillespie, W., Henry, D., O'Connell, D. and Robertson, J. (2000b) Vitamin D and vitamin D analogues for preventing fractures associated with involutional and post-menopausal osteoporosis. In *The Cochrane Library*, Issue 1. Oxford: Update Software.

Greenhalgh, T. (1997) *How to Read a Paper: The Basics of Evidence Based Medicine*. London: BMJ Publishing Group.

Guyatt, G. *et al.* (1993) Users' guides to the medical literature, II. How to use an article about therapy or prevention. A, Are the results of the study valid? *Journal of the American Medical Association*, 270(21), 2598–601.

Harden, A., Weston, R. and Oakley, A. (1999) *A Review of the Effectiveness and Appropriateness of Peer-delivered Health Promotion Interventions for Young People*. London: EPI-Centre, Social Science Research Unit.

Hey, V. (1994a) *Putting the Old in Their Place: Age, Ageing and Community Care*. London: Social Science Research Unit, Institute of Education University of London.

Hey, V. (1994b) *Elderly People, Choice and Community Care: A Report of a Research Project*. London: Headly Trust/Social Science Research Unit.

Hey, V. (1999) Frail elderly people: difficult questions and awkward answers. In S. Hood, B. Mayall and S. Oliver (eds) *Critical Issues in Social Research: Power and Prejudice*. Buckingham: Open University Press.

Lauritzen, J., Petersen, M. and Lund, B. (1993) Effect of external hip protectors on hip fractures. *Lancet*, 341, 11–13.

Milne, R., Donald, A. and Chambers, L. (1995) Piloting short workshops on the critical appraisal of reviews. *Health Trends*, 27(4), 120–3.

Milne, R. and Oliver, S. (1996) Evidence-based consumer health information: developing teaching in critical appraisal skills. *International Journal for Quality in Health Care*, 8(5), 439–45.

Oakley, A. (2000) *Experiments in Knowing: Gender and Method in the Social Sciences*. Cambridge: Polity Press.

Oliver, S., Nicholas, A. and Oakley, A. (1996) *Promoting Health after Sifting the Evidence (PHASE) Workshop Report*. London: EPI-Centre, Social Science Research Unit.

Oxman, A. *et al.* (1994) Users' guides to the medical literature, VI. How to use an overview. *Journal of the American Medical Association*, 272, 1367–71.

Parker, M., Gillespie, L. and Gillespie, W. (2000) Hip protectors for preventing hip fractures in the elderly. In *The Cochrane Library*, Issue 1. Oxford: Update Software.

See Tai, S., Parsons, T., Rutherford, O. and Iliffe, S. (2000) Physical activity for the prevention and treatment of osteoporosis in men. In *The Cochrane Library*, Issue 1. Oxford: Update Software.

Tugwell, P., Wells, G., Shea, B. *et al.* (2000) Hormone replacement therapy for osteoporosis in postmenopausal women. In *The Cochrane Library*, Issue 1. Oxford: Update Software.

WHO (1998) *The World Health Report 1998. Life in the 21st Century: A Vision for All.* Geneva: World Health Organization.

▶ **7**

▷ # Systematic reviews of effectiveness

▷ ## Greet Peersman, Sandy Oliver and Ann Oakley

Previous chapters have dealt with the need to consider evidence from sound research in the decision-making process about health promotion and public health interventions; the different types of research that need to be considered; and how research can be accessed and appraised for its validity, generalizability and applicability to the local context. The concept of a 'systematic review' was touched on as an important short-cut to accessing and integrating the findings from otherwise unmanageable amounts of, or sometimes hard to find, available primary research. This chapter discusses the key steps in conducting a systematic review and the barriers that need to be overcome if systematic reviews are to be used routinely in the decision-making process.

What makes a review systematic?

The answer lies in how the relevant primary research on a well defined topic is identified, appraised and synthesized, and in the reporting of these methods. The methods used in conducting a systematic review aim to limit both systematic errors (bias) and errors that occur by chance (random errors). These methods are explicitly reported so that others can assess the integrity of the review process and, hence, the validity of the review. The basic principles of systematic reviewing are the same, whatever the type of evidence considered, whether a review of randomized controlled trials (RCTs), observational studies, qualitative research or a combination of different types of research. For the purposes of this chapter, we mainly focus on reviewing 'effectiveness research', i.e. studies reporting the impact of health promotion interventions on health-related outcomes such as knowledge, attitudes, intentions, behaviour and health status. This focus does not imply that other types of research are redundant, but reflects the type of questions where systematic approaches are most advanced. The 'obsession' with trying to avoid errors and being explicit about how judgements were made throughout the review process is related to the potential use of systematic reviews in decisions about health care; decisions based on 'faulty' reviews can be misleading, or even harmful (Oxman 1994).

So what are the key steps in conducting a systematic review and to which errors is each step prone?

Formulating the review question

The first step is formulating the problem or subject matter the review will address. The purposes of reviews vary considerably: for example, to verify or develop theories; to size up substantive or methodological developments in a given field; to synthesize knowledge from different lines or fields of research; to infer generalizations about substantive issues; to formulate guidelines or legislation (Jackson 1980; Mulrow 1994). Being explicit about the aim of the review provides a frame of reference and helps to determine the types of studies and data to collect. A well conceived review addresses a precisely formulated question, rather than an ill-defined subject area (Mulrow 1987). Key components of a well formulated question for a review of effectiveness research are specifications of the study population, the types of interventions and the outcomes of interest (Mulrow and Oxman 1997). For example, 'Does school-based sex education (intervention) promote the initiation and/or frequency of sexual activity (outcomes) in young people (population)?'

The scope of the review question may be broad – for instance, in asking 'Which health promotion interventions reduce the risk of coronary heart disease in the general population?' – or relatively narrow, such as in the above school-based sex education example. In terms of the risk for bias, too narrow a focus may result in biased conclusions when the reviewer is familiar with the literature and narrows the scope of the review in such a way that studies that conflict with the reviewer's beliefs are excluded (Mulrow and Oxman 1997). Deciding the scope of the review in consultation with a range of potential users of the review may safeguard against this problem.

Though the review question should be clearly stated prior to embarking on the review, it may be subsequently refined in view of the evidence accumulated in the review process. However, data-driven review questions may generate spurious conclusions, and it is therefore important to be cautious about changing the review question in light of findings, and major changes are best avoided. If refinements are made, the appropriateness of the review methods – for instance, the search, the selection of studies or the data collection – should be reassessed, and any adjustments made (Mulrow and Oxman 1997).

Identifying relevant primary research

A comprehensive search is one of the key elements of a systematic review. The rationale is simple: 'what can be included in the review depends on what is found.' To minimize bias owing to inadequate searching, a variety of research sources need to be accessed, using strategies that are carefully developed and tested, and well documented. Chapter 4 deals with a range of available research sources, as well as with the complexities of developing an appropriate search strategy. Documenting the search strategies used in conducting a review is essential to enable others to replicate the process, as well as to enable them to assess whether the range of included studies represents the existing knowledge-base in a particular area, or whether it is likely that relevant studies have been missed. Potential bias is mainly related to missing studies that have not been published or have been published in non-English language journals; this is publication bias. Though there may be many reasons why researchers fail to publish their research findings, a well established problem is the under-representation of published studies showing no effect or even harmful effects (Simes 1986; Dickersin et al. 1987; Chalmers et al. 1993; Dickersin and Min 1993; Begg and Berlin 1998; Peersman et al. 1999a). Therefore, a special effort to identify unpublished studies is necessary. However, the resources provided for systematic reviews often do not allow for this labour-intensive and time-consuming activity. This could partly be overcome by ensuring that new reviews build on previously completed reviews which can be easily updated, an issue that is at the heart of the Cochrane Collaboration (see Chapter 1), and that is also taken up in more detail later on in this chapter.

Assessing identified studies for inclusion in the review

The next step is selecting the subset of studies for answering the review question out of the pool of studies that were identified by extensive searching. Searching on electronic databases, even with well developed search strategies, will result in a number of studies that do not fit within the boundaries of the review. This is because some of these studies share some of the terminology used in the search strategy or because there are inconsistencies in the indexing of research reports on those databases (Peersman et al. 1999b). Distinguishing between studies which are relevant within the context of the review and ones which are not requires the systematic application of explicit, predetermined, inclusion criteria. For effectiveness reviews,

these are often phrased in terms of the study population, the types of interventions, the outcomes of interest and specific research designs. Clearly,
they are based on and may extend the specifications in the review question.
Again, as with formulating the review question, inclusion criteria need to
be predetermined rather than *post hoc*, to prevent reviewers from describing
the studies *identified* rather than those they *aimed* to identify.

Selection of studies for inclusion in the review needs to be based on full
information about the study. In most cases, this means assessing the complete
written report, but sometimes it is also necessary to obtain additional information from the researchers who were involved in the study. In electronic
searching, only titles and/or abstracts are available in the first instance,
though more and more full reports are becoming available online. To
minimize bias, it is important to avoid assuming that a study is not relevant
based on incomplete information; more information needs to be gathered
before making a final decision. Failing to do so may exclude potentially
relevant studies from the review, which, in turn, may influence the findings.

Critically appraising studies meeting inclusion criteria

The next step is to appraise the studies critically in terms of their validity
(i.e. the extent to which their design and conduct are likely to prevent bias)
and certain design characteristics that affect interpretation of results (Mulrow
and Oxman 1997). The aim is to identify the subgroup of studies with
sufficient methodological strength to generate reliable conclusions on the
effectiveness of interventions. Well designed and well executed RCTs are
generally considered to provide the strongest evidence for an association
between the intervention tested and the change, if any, in health-related
outcomes in the study participants. Studies with less rigorous designs tend
to over-estimate the effectiveness of an intervention (i.e. erroneously concluding an intervention is effective) or provide less precise estimates of the
effect of an intervention (i.e. erroneously concluding no effect) (Chalmers
et al. 1983; Shulz *et al.* 1995; Mulrow and Oxman 1997; Peersman *et al.*
1999b). Attributing any changes in outcomes to the intervention under
study is particularly problematic in studies lacking a control or comparison
group (see also Chapter 2).

There are different potential sources of bias in trials, such as selection
bias, performance bias, attrition bias and detection bias. When people are
assigned to different study groups, the process needs to be impervious to
any influence by the individuals making the allocation, so that each individual has an equal chance to be assigned to the intervention or control/
comparison group. For instance, research findings would be misleading if
schools considered to be more amenable to working with a research team,
or in more needy areas, were more likely to be allocated to the intervention

group in a health promotion trial. Selection bias is most likely avoided if true random allocation (e.g. using random number tables) with adequate concealment (i.e. blinded randomization) is used (Mulrow and Oxman 1997). Performance bias relates to any systematic differences in the exposure to the interventions other than what was intended. For example, participants in the control group may be exposed to at least some of the intervention under study rather than no intervention at all (i.e. there is contamination between the groups), which may dilute the intervention effect. Attrition bias is introduced when there are systematic differences between those who drop out of a trial and those followed up for the duration of the trial; and/or differential drop-out between the different study groups. Bias can also occur when outcomes are assessed. Depending on the type of outcome assessment used, this could range from assessors being more likely to record changes in the intervention group than the control or comparison group when they know which group individuals belong to, to doubts about the validity of outcome measures used. In addition to problems with the assignment and execution of a trial, there may also be problems with how the data were analysed, such as using inappropriate statistical techniques, or how the data were reported, such as selective reporting of only those outcomes for which a positive intervention effect was found.

Since there is no strong empirical evidence of a relationship between trial outcomes and specific criteria used to assess the risk of different biases and other threats to the validity or reliability of the study findings, there is no set of widely agreed criteria for assessing the 'quality' of studies (Mulrow and Oxman 1997; Peersman et al. 1999a, b). (Indeed, applying a range of checklists to the same set of studies can lead to very different estimates of effectiveness: Juni et al. 1999). Hence, different systematic reviews use different sets of criteria. For example, the EPPI-Centre assesses the quality of outcome evaluation studies by noting the presence or absence of eight methodological criteria which are related to each of the above discussed risks for bias at the selection, execution and analysis stages of the study. They were derived from quality criteria recommended by other authors of systematic reviews in health promotion (Schaps et al. 1981; Loevinsohn 1990) and from a methodological study conducted as part of a school-based RCT of smoking prevention (Biglan et al. 1987a, b). The eight criteria are: (a) clear definition of the aims of the intervention; (b) description of the intervention content and the evaluation design sufficiently detailed to allow replication; (c) the use of random allocation to the different groups, including the control/comparison group(s), resulting in equivalent groups in terms of socio-demographic and baseline outcome variables; (d) provision of numbers of participants recruited to each group; (e) provision of pre-intervention outcome data for each group; (f) provision of post-intervention outcome data for each group; (g) attrition reported for each group; (h) findings reported for each outcome measure targeted as indicated in the aims of the study.

Applying these criteria to 112 outcome evaluations of the effectiveness of sexual health promotion interventions for young people (Peersman *et al.* 1996), we found that: most studies (86 per cent) clearly stated the aims of the intervention; only 31 per cent used random allocation to the different groups involved; 60 per cent provided enough information to replicate the intervention; 58 per cent gave the numbers recruited; 43 per cent provided pre-intervention data; 42 per cent discussed the problem of attrition; 43 per cent provided post-intervention data for all the groups in the study; and 84 per cent discussed the impact on all the outcomes specified as targets of the intervention. Perhaps it is not surprising that the use of random allocation was relatively low, but it is disappointing how many studies did not state how many people they actually included.

Incorporating assessments of study quality in reviews

There are several ways in which the above 'quality' assessments can be used in a review. For example, reviewers may decide to set a cut-off point for including studies based on meeting certain quality criteria. In the review of 112 studies of sexual health promotion interventions, studies having all eight criteria are deemed 'gold standard' evaluations; those with a subset of four criteria are regarded as 'sound' evaluations. These are criteria (a), (e), (f) and (h). For criterion (c) non-random allocation was included, and an exception was made for criterion (e) in the case of a Solomon four-group design (this is a design that includes two additional control groups to assess the effect, if any, of testing *per se*) (Campbell and Stanley 1963). The four 'minimum standard' criteria were chosen in recognition of the fact that non-randomized trials are not necessarily worse than randomized trials, but that baseline equivalence is crucial; that it is essential to be able to judge the effect, if any, of the intervention; and that authors often neglect to report on those outcomes for which no effect or even a harmful effect was noted, which may skew the conclusions of the study. Ten (9 per cent) of the 112 studies of the sexual health review met the eight 'gold standard' methodological criteria and an additional 13 met the four 'minimum standard' criteria. Only 10 (29 per cent) of the 35 RCTs were assessed as 'gold standard' and 17 (49 per cent) as 'sound'. The main methodological problem with the RCTs not judged to be 'sound' was a failure to report pre-intervention (78 per cent) and post-intervention data (67 per cent). Overall, 89 (79 per cent) studies failed to meet the minimum criteria for a 'sound' study, with the implication that the conclusions about effectiveness presented by the authors could not be treated as reliable. A final element in the EPPI-Centre reviewing process consisted of comparing the reviewers' assessments of effectiveness with those provided by the authors themselves: overall, most (93; 87 per cent) studies reported that the experimental interventions were effective in changing at least one of the outcomes targeted. For the 23 sound outcome evaluations, there was 52 per cent agreement between authors and reviewers on the interventions being effective for at least one of the outcomes targeted; eight per cent agreement on their effectiveness for some groups only; and four per cent agreement as to some positive effect. In 34 per cent of cases, authors judged the intervention effective but the reviewers disagreed; the reviewers judged these interventions ineffective or unclear in their effect, suggesting that authors' conclusions about effectiveness were not necessarily reliable, even if the evaluation study was judged to be 'sound'. Disagreement between authors and reviewers was mainly owing to authors over-stating an intervention effect that was not statistically significant as noted from the data presented.

Extracting relevant data

Following selection of a set of studies that meet the criteria for relevance and validity of their findings, the next step is to extract detailed information on the study population; the intervention content, delivery and setting; and any other characteristics of the study that may be related to the observed changes, if any, in the outcomes targeted. For this purpose, a sensible strategy is to develop a standardized data collection form to ensure that similar information is collected from each study and thus the characteristics of studies can be compared on equal terms, and to be explicit about the multitude of decisions that occur throughout the review process, including the validity assessments explained above. An example of such a data abstraction form, the EPPI-Centre Review Guidelines (Peersman et al. 1997), is available on the EPPI-Centre's website (http://eppi.ioe.ac.uk/). Though primarily developed for collecting data from outcome evaluation studies for the purpose of synthesizing findings across different studies, this tool can also be used to analyse an individual study, or as a checklist for writing a research report to ensure that reporting on the study is thorough. The EPPI-Centre review guidelines consist of seven major sections. The first section collects bibliographic information about the study: the authors, the title of the report, whether it was published or not and where, the report date and language, where and how it was found. Section two deals with the support for the study: the source of funding and the contact details of the first author of the report in case any clarification or missing data need to be obtained. Then the type of evaluation study (process and/or outcome evaluation; retrospective versus prospective) is noted. Subsequent sections of the guidelines are completed as appropriate. These form the bulk of the data collection and record, in as much detail as is reported, the planning, content, delivery and implementation of the intervention(s), as well as the study population characteristics, the methodological quality of the study and its evaluation findings. Definitions of terminology used and instructions for making key decisions (e.g. is the outcome evaluation 'sound'?) are specified throughout. To minimize errors in the data abstraction process, it is generally considered good practice for two reviewers to gather data on each study independently, and for the data sets to be compared. In this way, any errors can be caught, such as overlooking relevant information in the study report or misinterpreting information provided. Any discrepancies between the two independent data sets are then resolved by consensus in discussion between the reviewers, if necessary with the input from a third reviewer. This is not a trivial issue; the way in which the research reports are written is highly variable and the quality of reporting key information is often poor, presenting considerable challenges to the reviewers (and any reader of such reports). Careful investigations of 'double reviewing' have concluded that discrepancies are almost inevitable and continued vigilence and discussion of discrepancies is essential (Strang *et al.* 1997; Floyd *et al.* 1998).

The data abstraction process results in a potentially huge data set, depending on the number of studies considered. An efficient data management system is therefore required. These days this means a computerized database, such as the one developed by the EPPI-Centre referred to as EPIC. This not only helps reviewers with data collection, verification and analysis, but also provides an important dissemination tool (discussed in more detail below; see also Chapter 3).

Analysing and presenting results

The most essential element of an analysis is a thoughtful approach that considers: the comparisons that should be made in relation to the review question or hypotheses posed; what study results should be use in each comparison; whether the results are similar within each comparison; what the best summary effect for each comparison is; and how reliable those summaries are (Mulrow and Oxman 1997). Statistical methods for combining the results of different studies (meta-analysis) may be used, but it is not always possible to use these (due to lack of relevant, valid data) and this approach is not necessarily appropriate (it may combine study results in misleading ways) (Mulrow and Oxman 1997).

Interpreting results

The way a review is done affects its findings (Peersman *et al.* 1999b). Because there are different approaches to conducting a systematic review, it is important to consider assessing how sensitive the results are to changes in some of the key decisions and assumptions that were made during the review process. Examples of such sensitivity analyses are: including or excluding studies where there is some ambiguity as to whether they meet the inclusion criteria; re-analysing the data using a reasonable range of values for missing data; and excluding unpublished studies (Oxman 1994).

The primary aim of the discussion and conclusions of the review is to help people to understand the implications of the evidence in relationship to practical decisions (Mulrow and Oxman 1997). Though the conclusions of a review should not exceed the evidence that is reviewed, it is helpful to discuss how the evidence from included studies fits into the context of other evidence. However, it is impossible for reviews to provide all the information that is needed for people making decisions.

Facilitating the use of systematic reviews

Though there has been increasing enthusiasm in health care and health promotion for conducting systematic reviews, they have not always been well received by potential users, especially health promotion practitioners. Some have criticized the over-simplification of health promotion interventions, considered to be complex in nature and effect, for the purpose of being able to communicate the research findings and implications. Others have targeted the misuse of the 'medical paradigm', with its focus on methodological rigour of the evaluation rather than the appropriateness of the intervention (Health Education Board for Scotland 1996).

To explore how effectiveness reviews could be improved to address the information needs better, the EPPI-Centre convened two consultation meetings in 1999 with commissioners, purchasers and providers of health promotion services. The discussions centred on the nature of effectiveness reviews and what were considered to be important elements of effectiveness reviews.

Participants appreciated the explicit and transparent methodology used in systematic reviews: a full discussion and critical appraisal of the study findings, including discrepancies, but not value judgements. They emphasized the need for sufficient detail in the descriptions of the interventions and the quality of the resources or training of the provider involved in the intervention. Process data were also highlighted as important in complementing the information about the effectiveness of an intervention in terms of how the intervention may have worked or why it may have failed to work. A summary of the review which incorporates clear 'bottom line' implications for planning services and identifying gaps in knowledge was considered essential.

Avoiding disappointment with the end-product was considered crucial. More clarity in advance about the information needs of potential users of reviews should minimize disappointment with the final product, and involving end-users of reviews in various stages of the review process was considered a good strategy to that effect. However, competing information needs do occur. While research commissioners felt the need for broad reviews to answer policy-related questions, practitioners felt they needed more intervention-specific information. Practitioners often have very specific questions about 'what works'; they have ideas about the interventions they wish to provide, and would like the evidence about these specific interventions presented. An additional problem is that effectiveness reviews that are largely shaped by the available evaluation literature have not always been explicitly linked with current practice. Practitioners would find it, for example, most useful to have systematic reviews of 'approaches' to health promotion (e.g. community development or peer-delivered interventions), rather than topic-focused reviews (e.g. healthy eating or accident prevention).

Participants emphasized the role of the UK government in the dissemination of systematic reviews, and that partnerships were required to make different products aimed at different audiences possible; for example, practitioners writing for practitioners. Because practitioners often need to seek out evidence of effectiveness for themselves, information about effective search strategies should be disseminated and training in critical appraisal skills supported. However, an important reason why reviews or research evidence are not used in service planning, is that other constraints, such as political pressures, determine decisions.

It is clear that several problems need to be addressed if systematic reviews are to be used more routinely in programme planning and policy-making. Some of those, such as the need for more detailed information about the intervention content, delivery and implementation, also need to be addressed at the level of the primary research report. Often, however, the word limit for journal submissions constrains researchers in documenting this information. Alternative routes for dissemination of programme manuals can help to overcome this problem. For example, some researchers refer readers to documents posted on the Web. Incorporating clear 'bottom line' implications for planning services and identifying gaps in knowledge is often hindered by the fact that the research evidence is insufficient to give clear answers or recommendations. Further improvement in the design and evaluation of interventions will make an important contribution to advancing the knowledge base in health promotion. The need to link the focus of systematic reviews more closely to current practice is an important one. Systematic reviews often lag behind innovations in the field. Part of the problem is the relative lack of evaluation studies of innovative interventions in the public domain. Often, interventions are not evaluated due to lack of resources, or results are not disseminated (Health Education Board for Scotland 1996). In addition, systematic reviews are too often commissioned as 'one-off' exercises. Given the labour-intensive and time-consuming process of conducting a systematic review, especially one with a broad scope, it is essential that new reviews build on earlier reviews to meet information needs in a timely fashion. For example, EPIC, developed by the EPPI-Centre, is a cumulative database of studies. Depending on the focus of the commissioned review, only data from studies that meet the specific relevance criteria for the review are entered in the database. However, the *types* of data collected (i.e. characteristics of the intervention content, delivery and implementation, the study population and the evaluation findings) are the same for each review, irrespective of its particular focus. All such data are entered in EPIC, which has now become a repository of data on approximately 500 evaluation studies of interventions in different areas of health promotion (e.g. workplace health promotion, sexual health promotion, mental health promotion). This not only allows for the efficient updating of topic-related reviews with new research studies, it also allows for the synthesis of studies with common characteristics – for example, the delivery methods – across different areas of health promotion. The 'peer education' review discussed in Chapter 8 is a good example; it pulls together the findings on the effectiveness of peer education for young people from studies conducted in different areas of health promotion. The review was able to draw on some studies in the EPIC database which had already been reviewed as part of a topic-related review of sexual health promotion studies.

All this activity is wasted if the results of systematic reviews are not disseminated widely and in an appropriate way to different audiences. Systematic reviews conducted by the Cochrane Collaboration are disseminated as part of 'the Cochrane Library' on CD-ROM as well as on-line (http://update.cochrane.co.uk). This resource currently contains over 800 completed reviews in different areas of health care (the Cochrane Database of Systematic Reviews, CDSR), as well as structured abstracts of more than 1,700 other good quality systematic reviews from around the world (the York Database of Abstracts of Reviews of Effectiveness, DARE), the Cochrane Controlled Trials Register (CCTR) of over 250,000 citations of controlled trials and a bibliography of articles on systematic review methods (the Cochrane Review Methodology Database, CRMD). Other sources for good quality reviews are the technology assessments (DEC Reports) of the Wessex Institute of Public Health (http://cochrane.epi.bris.ac.uk/rd) and the systematic reviews produced within the UK National Health Service Research and Development Programme (http://www.update-software.com/national/). A register of over 400 effectiveness reviews specific to health promotion can be found on the EPPI-Centre website at http://eppi.ioe.ac.uk/; this includes both systematic and traditional literature reviews. This number of reviews is surprising, and the apparent duplication of effort and variable quality is disappointing (see also Chapter 3).

The overall aim of systematic reviews is to facilitate the use of critically appraised evidence in the planning of new health promotion services and research, whether at a national level or within a local context. The challenge is to come up with a system that is responsive to the many and diverse information needs. In addition to the dissemination of its systematic reviews in printed format, the EPPI-Centre is also experimenting with making the EPIC database of evaluation studies available for public use. The advantage of EPIC is that in addition to being able to pool findings across different studies, the database can be searched for individual studies that are relevant to answering more specific questions (see also Chapter 3). For example: 'In what ways can workplace health promotion involve the target population in the design and evaluation of successful interventions?'; or 'Which sexual health promotion studies have employed outreach methods to access out-of-school young people, and what types of interventions have been successful within this setting?' Though a lot of progress has been made in assimilating a reliable knowledge-base and encouraging people to use it in decision-making, a continued and concerted effort is needed.

Conclusions

The key messages from this chapter are:

- The basic principles of systematic reviewing are the same, whatever the type of evidence considered.
- Being explicit about how a review was carried out and what has been included helps readers to decide whether the review is valid and useful for them.
- Collaboration with other reviewers and with potential users of reviews is essential in avoiding duplication of effort and keeping reviews relevant and current with new available evidence.
- Reviews are useful if they resonate with questions from the broad practice of the health promotion field.

References

Begg, C. and Berlin, J. (1988) Publication bias: a problem in interpreting medical data. *Journal of the Royal Statistical Society*, 151, 419–63.

Biglan, A., Glasgow, R., Ary, D. *et al.* (1987a). How generalisable are the effects of smoking prevention programs? Refusal skills training and parent messages in a teacher-administered program. *Journal of Behavioral Medicine*, 10(6), 613–28.

Biglan, A., Severson, H., Ary, D. *et al.* (1987b) Do smoking prevention programs really work? Attrition and the internal and external validity of an evaluation of a refusal skills training program. *Journal of Behavioral Medicine*, 10(2), 159–71.

Campbell, D. and Stanley, J. (1963) *Experimental and Quasi-experimental Designs for Research*. Chicago: Rand-McNally.

Chalmers, T., Celano, P., Sacks, H. and Smith, H. Jr (1983) Bias in treatment assignment in controlled clinical trials. *New England Journal of Medicine*, 309(22), 1358–61.

Chalmers, I., Enkin, M. and Keirse, M. (1993) Preparing and updating systematic reviews of randomized controlled trials of health care. *The Milbank Quarterly*, 71, 411–33.

Dickersin, K., Chan, S., Chalmers, T. and Sacks, H. Jr (1987) Publication bias and clinical trials. *Controlled Clinical Trials*, 8, 343–53.

Dickersin, K. and Min, Y. (1993) NIH clinical trials and publication bias. *Online Journal of Current Clinical Trials* (serial online), Doc. no. 50.

Floyd, J. A., Moulton, R. A. and Medler, S. M. (1998) Effective intercoder reliability for systematic reviews. Paper presented at the Sixth Annual Cochrane Colloquium, Baltimore, October.

Health Education Board for Scotland, Research and Evaluation Division (1996) How effective are effectiveness reviews? *Health Education Journal*, 55, 359–62.

Jackson, G. (1980) Methods for integrative reviews. *Review of Educational Research*, 50(3), 438–60.

Juni, P., Witschi, A., Bloch, R. and Egger, M. (1999) The hazards of scoring the quality of clinical trials for meta-analysis. *JAMA*, 282(11), 1054–60.

Loevinsohn, B. (1990) Health education interventions in developing countries: a methodological review of published articles. *International Journal of Epidemiology*, 4, 788–94.

Mulrow, C. (1987) The medical review article: state of the science. *Annals of Internal Medicine*, 106, 485–8.

Mulrow, C. (1994) Rationale for systematic reviews. *British Medical Journal*, 309, 597–9.

Mulrow, C. and Oxman, A. (1997) *How to Conduct a Cochrane Systematic Review*. San Antonio: Cochrane Collaboration.

Oxman, A. (1994) Checklists for review articles. *British Medical Journal*, 309, 648–51.

Peersman, G., Harden, A., Oliver, S. and Oakley, A. (1999a) *Effectiveness Reviews in Health Promotion*. London: EPI-Centre, Social Science Research Unit.

Peersman, G., Harden, A., Oliver, S. and Oakley, A. (1999b) Discrepancies in findings from effectiveness reviews: the case of health promotion interventions to change cholesterol levels. *Health Education Journal*, 58, 192–202.

Peersman, G., Oakley, A., Oliver, S. and Thomas, T. (1996) *Review of Effectiveness of Sexual Health Promotion Interventions for Young People*. London: EPI-Centre, Social Science Research Unit.

Peersman, G., Oliver, S. and Oakley, A. (1997) *Review Guidelines. Data Collection for the EPIC Database*. London: EPI-Centre, Social Science Research Unit

Schaps, E., DiBartolo, R., Moskowitz, J. *et al.* (1981) A review of 127 drug abuse prevention program evaluations. *Journal of Drug Issues*, 11(1), 17–43.

Shulz, K., Chalmers, I., Hayes, R. and Altman, D. (1995) Empirical evidence of bias: dimensions of methodological quality associated with estimates of treatment effects in controlled trials. *Journal of the American Medical Association*, 273(5), 408–12.

Simes, R. (1986) Publication bias: the case for an international registry of clinical trials. *Journal of Clinical Oncology*, 4, 1529–41.

Strang, W. N., Boissel, P. and Uberla, K. (1997) Inter-reader variation. Paper presented to the Second International Conference, Scientific Basis of Health Services and Fifth Annual Cochrane Colloquium, Amsterdam, October.

▶ **Part 3**

▷ Applying health promotion and research to young people's lives

▶ 8

▷ The fine detail: conducting a systematic review

▷ Angela Harden

So far, the chapters in this book have outlined the rationale, the 'how-to' and some of the debates surrounding using research for informing decision-making in health promotion. More specifically, they have introduced the value of conducting systematic reviews within health promotion. But what is it like actually to conduct a systematic review? How do the issues raised in previous chapters affect the methods used to conduct the review and the final review 'product'? For example, one of the issues raised in Chapter 4 was the difficulty of conducting an exhaustive search of the literature. In the course of a systematic review, what might be the implication of having limited resources to search the literature? This chapter provides an insight into the practicalities of 'doing' systematic reviews by using a recently completed systematic review as a case study: a review of the effectiveness and appropriateness of peer-delivered health promotion for young people (Harden *et al.* 1999a). This illustrates how systematic reviews can balance the need to apply rigorous research methods with the need for a review that will be relevant and applicable in practice.

Setting priorities and defining methods for a systematic review

In August 1998, as part of a three-year programme of work at the EPPI-Centre funded by the Department of Health in the UK, a brief proposal was submitted for a systematic review of the effectiveness and appropriateness of peer-delivered health promotion for young people. This brief proposal was submitted as part of a 'menu' of choices for policy makers of six different systematic reviews of health promotion. At this time no systematic review on this method of health promotion existed. This was a significant gap, as the method was becoming hugely popular and was being widely used in numerous health promotion projects around the UK, Europe and worldwide, and great claims were being made regarding both its efficacy and its potential to engage young people actively in promoting their own and others health (Milburn 1995; Wilton *et al.* 1995; Svenson 1998). In the UK, the Department of Health had already funded a pilot study for a randomized controlled trial of peer-led sex education (Charleston *et al.* 1996) and the full trial, funded by the Medical Research Council, was currently under way (see Chapter 11 for a discussion of this trial). Thus, from a policy and research point of view, there was an urgent need for a review that could synthesize the existing research on peer-delivered health promotion, and we were asked to draw up a full proposal for the review.

As systematic reviews are intended to help to bridge the gap between research and practice, it is important to ensure that reviews are addressing relevant practice questions in a way that will produce relevant findings. Systematic reviews commissioned by the NHS Health Technology Assessment programme, for example, explicitly aim to ensure that high-quality information on the costs, effectiveness and broader impact of health technologies is produced in the most economical way for those who *use, manage* and *provide care* in the NHS. This is achieved by involving practitioners, managers, users and researchers in identifying and prioritizing research topics and refining research questions before research is commissioned, and in commenting on the findings before they are published (Oliver *et al.* 2001). Researchers seeking funds outside of such systems – for instance, when applying to responsive research programmes – need to be proactive in taking into account broader views when proposing reviews. Where the views of potential users have clearly informed a proposal, it is less likely to fail at the stage of 'peer refereeing' when research funders ask other experts to comment on the likely usefulness of the research.

Developing the review proposal

In terms of our review, at this stage we knew that it would be addressing both policy and research questions. We also needed to be proactive in addressing the questions of practitioners. To do this we drew on two sources of information: the debate on effectiveness reviews in the research and practice literature and our own consultations with practitioners. Published debates criticized systematic reviews of health promotion literature for transplanting inappropriate methods from systematic reviews of the effects of health care. Our own consultations with practitioners echoed these criticisms (Oliver *et al.* 1996; Peersman *et al.* 1998; see Chapter 7 for a fuller discussion). This led to a lack of concrete recommendations for practice owing to a small evidence base and the mismatch between the kinds of interventions evaluated in the studies included in reviews and those interventions actually implemented in UK practice. One of the main ways forward for systematic reviews offered by review users was the importance of getting the balance right between the need for rigorous research to establish the effectiveness of health promotion and the need to make reviews relevant to practice. Suggested ways of doing this were the inclusion of process as well as outcome data and full discussion and critical appraisal of findings from the review.

With this in mind, the proposal for the review featured several significant elements designed to help us focus on questions of relevance to potential end-users of the review. We had already addressed some concerns in setting the review: it did not focus on a specific health problem but on an approach to promoting health. In addition, the review explicitly aimed to include outcome evaluations, in order to examine the effectiveness of peer-delivered health promotion, and process evaluations, in order to examine the appropriateness of this method. In answering the question of appropriateness, we considered the acceptability of peer-delivered interventions compared with those delivered by professionals or other adults. In other words, how did young people value the approach? We examined how peer-delivered interventions were working or not working (e.g. what factors are related to successful implementation?). Finally, we prepared the review in two stages, with a meeting with potential end-users of the review (policy makers, service providers and other researchers) after an exhaustive search and descriptive mapping of the relevant research literature was complete. These potential users were then able to consider and recommend those analyses they might find most useful after discussing a completed research mapped according to its key characteristics (for instance, the number of outcome or process evaluations, in which health areas, implementing which 'models' of peer-delivered health promotion). There were thus two distinct stages to the overall review: a descriptive mapping and an 'in-depth' review of a subset of studies from the mapping. The time scale and resources for the review were set over a nine-month period with the equivalent of two full-time researchers.

Revising the proposed methods of the review

The proposal was sent to three referees by the Department of Health who represented 'experts' in health promotion research, policy and practice. Not all the referees considered the proposed review a priority. For example, one referee questioned the need for the review altogether and suggested that the method was not popular in current practice, while the other two very much supported and welcomed it. The same referee suggested that it would be valuable to examine the transferability of peer education to other age groups. While all referees welcomed our intention to include process as well as outcome evaluations, they suggested we tighten some of our definitions and be more explicit at various stages of the review. Stressing the diversity of peer-delivered approaches available, all referees emphasized the need for us to look at the different theoretical models and assumptions underlying this approach (e.g. the definition of 'peer', whether the approach is driven by young people or adults, how the approach fits in with others, such as community education). We therefore decided to pay particular attention to coding such diversity in our initial descriptive mapping and in the analysis of our findings. All the referees were confused by our proposed procedures for differently assessing the quality of process and outcome evaluations, and later reports were more explicit.

Clearly, balancing the differing views of potential users of the review was a challenge and it was impossible to act on all suggestions. But by eliciting their views we had at least been made aware of what they were. We could then be explicit about the views we had not considered and discuss these as part of the potential limitations of the review. We could not, however, be explicit about the views of groups of people we had not consulted. For example, a key group of people in this respect was young people themselves. Groups of young people who may have been key stakeholders in the context of this review might have been those who had experience of being a peer educator or those who had received peer education.

The processes of a systematic review

As outlined in Chapter 7, the key features of a systematic review are that efforts are made to assure quality at each stage in the review process and the methods used in the review are explicitly reported so that others are able to judge the validity of the review findings. This section of the chapter illustrates how we attempted to assure quality and rigour within the context of the various resource constraints of the review, while keeping in mind the need to consider user demands for relevance. This involved mixing well rehearsed methods in systematic reviewing with new methodological developments.

Searching the literature

To be exhaustive in our search for research on peer-delivered health promotion, we searched bibliographic databases and sources of quality-assessed research literature, and used handsearching, personal contacts and scanning of the reference lists of already identified relevant research reports (see Chapter 4). One of the first challenges that confronted us was translating what we wanted to find into search strategies to use on bibliographic databases. Using research that we had already identified, we knew that some reports did not use terms such as 'peer education' to describe an intervention which had been delivered to young people by young people. We therefore had to anticipate many alternative terms. Further, although some databases had specific controlled vocabulary terms that captured the concept of using peers to deliver education (for example, PsycLIT and ERIC provided the term 'peer counselling' or 'peer-tutoring'), others did not. In addition to these controlled vocabulary terms, we therefore also had to use approximately 70 'free-text' terms to capture all the different ways that interventions delivered by peers might be described in a title or abstract (e.g. 'peer-led', 'delivered by young people', 'implemented by teens').

As bibliographic databases and handsearching are not very good for locating unpublished literature, we knew that we had to seek out unpublished literature. This was particularly welcomed by our three referees. All of them emphasized the importance of accessing unpublished reports in terms of increasing the review's chances of including interventions that are actually in current practice. As these are more likely to have been evaluated by practitioners, who are less likely to publish their research, the referees argued that it would be important to invest resources in tracking this research down. We used the specialized health promotion databases of the Health Education Authority (England) and Health Education Board (Scotland) and a specialized journal (*Xcellent: the Journal of Peer Education in Scotland*) to track down unpublished literature. Once identified we then wrote to individual practitioners or organizations to obtain copies of the full reports. This special effort paid off: we identified 25 unpublished reports, and five of these (representing 30 per cent of all the process evaluations included in the review) were able to contribute to the review's conclusions and recommendations.

Mapping the literature

In total, our searches yielded 5,124 citations, of which 421 were reports that discussed, described or evaluated peer-delivered health promotion for young people aged 11 to 24. While studies which discussed or reviewed the literature on this topic would form the background to the review, we knew that we were only interested in reviewing the part of the literature which evaluated either the effectiveness of peer-delivered health promotion (outcome evaluations) or the appropriateness (process evaluations). Given the time scale for the review, we knew that it would be impossible to review all 172 outcome evaluations and 82 process-only evaluations in-depth. We thus needed to set some priorities.

To help to set these priorities the 421 reports were categorized in order to map research activity according to study type, country in which the study was carried out, health focus, population characteristics and, for studies reporting on interventions, intervention site, provider and type using the EPPI-Centre health promotion keywording strategy (Peersman and Oliver 1997; for a fuller discussion of this strategy, see Chapter 3). Taking on board the reviewers' comments about the diversity of approaches within peer-delivered health promotion, we also keyworded reports which described or evaluated an intervention according to: whether the intervention was based on the self-defined needs of young people themselves; whether it was developed in partnership with young people; the age of the peer-leaders; and the theoretical model on which the intervention was based. In terms of the effectiveness of peer-delivered health promotion, we also wanted to know which studies would potentially be able to provide us with the most reliable evidence. We thus undertook a quality screening exercise of the outcome evaluations. Those that had employed a control or comparison group (demonstrated to be equivalent to the intervention group) and had reported both pre- and post-intervention data were classified as 'potentially sound'.

Developing inclusion criteria: selecting studies for in-depth review

From the mapping and quality screening exercise we were able to suggest several criteria for in-depth review. As the reviewers of our proposal and we had anticipated, there was enormous diversity among the interventions. While such diversity would be valuable in identifying patterns of effective/ ineffective, appropriate/inappropriate interventions, it was questionable whether it was possible to include very different types of interventions in the same review, as they seemed to be doing something qualitatively different from other types. For example, in some interventions, peer leaders were used to deliver only one component of a multi-component intervention and we were concerned about whether such an intervention warranted classification as peer-delivered health promotion. The inclusion of 'peer counselling' interventions, in which young people are trained to respond to and help other young people to deal with their immediate personal problems, were also considered to be qualitatively different from peer-delivered health promotion aimed at whole groups or communities. As we had identified a large number of evaluations of this type of intervention it would be more sensible to recommend that a separate systematic review be commissioned, rather than trying to handle them in the current review. We therefore prioritized certain 'types' of peer-delivered health promotion, including those which used young people as the sole providers of an intervention and those which provided interventions for groups of young people rather than particular individuals in need. Although it was difficult to make the decision to exclude these studies from the in-depth review, we felt that by doing so it would be easier to interpret the findings of the review. As noted above, we had also coded outcome evaluations according to their quality. We felt that given our resources for synthesizing the evidence on effectiveness we should prioritize good-quality outcome evaluations. For process-only evaluations, however, we included any study that had clearly described methods and results.

Our priority setting had so far been informed by referees' comments on our initial proposal, our descriptive mapping of the literature and the need to base conclusions and recommendations on research of a high quality. To be sure that we were not way off track with these, we decided to present the results of the descriptive mapping and quality screening exercise to the EPPI-Centre health promotion steering group. This group consisted of representatives from the practitioner, researcher and policy-making groups and includes those with specialist knowledge in health promotion and/or systematic review methods. This group felt strongly that the mapping had been useful in highlighting commonalities and differences in interventions and had helped to determine more specific review questions and feasible review products. They also reaffirmed our decision to include process evaluations as well as high-quality outcome evaluations.

Data extraction and quality assessment

After applying our inclusion criteria we had 49 outcome evaluations and 15 process evaluations from which to extract data. The same set of detailed data was needed from each study. Superficial and inconsistent data extraction from studies risks the studies being used inaccurately, inconsistently and in vague, unspecified ways. Conclusions drawn on such an approach would be largely subjective and could be very misleading. Our review proposal specified two researchers independently using a set of standardized guidelines (Peersman et al. 1997; see http://eppi.ioe.ac.uk/) to extract data and critically to appraise process and outcome evaluations. Although labour-intensive, double reviewing had huge benefits: systematic and 'random' errors were more likely to be eliminated; it weeded out ambiguity, as reviewers were obliged to explain their categorization and interpretation to each other; it helped reviewers to identify and be reflective about their own subjective biases; and the in-depth discussion between two reviewers led to more creative thinking.

This last benefit particularly applied to areas that were generally not reported very well, such as issues surrounding who made the decisions about why a particular intervention was implemented and how it was to be evaluated. For example, the two reviewers often disagreed on issues related to how the intervention was developed (e.g. whether an intervention was based on a needs assessment and, if so, what type; whether the intervention developed according to a theoretical model). There were times when this was the result of an oversight on the part of one reviewer. However, at other times it reflected the differences in the knowledge base and experience the two reviewers brought to the study (one had a background in psychology, the other in education), and through discussion a better understanding and way of conceptualizing the processes that had been used to develop the intervention were arrived at.

One of the biggest challenges for this stage of the review related to our decision to include process evaluations as well as outcome evaluations. Process evaluations can use a variety of study designs and methods of data collection, such as cross-sectional surveys, observation or in-depth interviews. Although there is no absolute consensus on criteria for assessing the quality of studies that are designed to measure the effectiveness of interventions, agreed criteria do exist (e.g. Chalmers et al. 1989; MacDonald et al. 1992; for a fuller discussion see Peersman et al. 1998). However, this is not the case for other types of study designs and methods of data collection. We decided to draw on the criteria proposed by four research groups (Cobb and Hagemaster, 1987; Mays and Pope, 1995; Boulton et al. 1996; Medical Sociology Group 1996) to assess the validity and reliability of 'qualitative' research, as presented in Oakley (2000).

The criteria required the reviewers to make judgements about the clarity of the aims, context, sample and methodology; and the sufficiency of data for linking evidence and interpretation. These criteria and the consequences of applying them are discussed more fully in Chapter 2. However, it is worth briefly reflecting here on some of the challenges of this process. Many of these involved the difficulties the two reviewers had in applying the criteria in the most standardized way possible. The original research groups gave no guidance for what exactly constituted 'clear' or 'sufficient', and this posed a problem for trying to negotiate a shared definition between the two reviewers and between studies. Overall, the agreement for the two reviewers in applying the quality criteria ranged from 87 per cent for 'inclusion of sufficient original data to mediate between data and interpretation' to 60 per cent for 'clear description of sample'. To reach agreement, the reviewers had to look not only to themselves to resolve disagreement (in terms of differences in research and other professional experience), but also across all the studies. For example, both reviewers had high expectations of what should constitute a report having provided a 'clear' description of the sample. However, we were soon having to make relative judgements, as such detail was often at best minimal and at worst completely lacking.

Synthesizing the findings and drawing recommendations

After extracting data and quality assessing the outcome evaluations, we had 12 soundly evaluated interventions from which to draw recommendations about effectiveness. We also had the findings from the 16 process-only evaluations that we had included in the in-depth review. Although at first sight these might seem to be very small numbers, they were in line with other systematic reviews of health promotion and do not necessarily pre-clude being able to make recommendations. Synthesis of the findings from both types of studies (outcome evaluations and process evaluations) started with a detailed narrative description of each study.

In terms of synthesizing the findings of these studies about effectiveness, it was very obvious that we would not be able to use meta-analysis, as the interventions and the way they had been evaluated varied greatly. We thus had to synthesize the findings in a purely 'narrative' form. As highlighted in Chapter 7, there are few specific guidelines for how to synthesize findings when meta-analysis is not possible and even fewer for drawing up recom-mendations. However, we were able to build on the way we had synthes-ized findings and drawn up recommendations in previous EPPI-Centre systematic reviews (e.g. Oakley *et al.* 1995; Peersman *et al.* 1996; Harden *et al.* 1999b), and by reflecting on the processes we went through, several 'procedures' emerged. Overarching all procedures was a commitment to trying to make explicit how we were making judgements and drawing re-commendations. We first looked very generally and found that more studies found peer-delivered health promotion to be effective than ineffective. From these we were able to recommend that 'Professionals involved in the pro-motion of young people's health can choose from a pool of several different interventions' (Harden *et al.* 1999a: 4), while being very specific about the potential limitations in the generalizability or transferability of interven-tions. For example,

> School-based smoking prevention interventions, targeted at 11 to 13 year olds, which use the same-age or older peer leaders to teach skills to resist peer and other social pressures, have been demonstrated to be effective. However, these positive effects may not be generalisable to all groups of young people, especially those who are at higher risk of smoking in the future.
>
> (Harden *et al.* 1999a: 4)

We then went on to note that none of the studies showed that peer leaders were less effective than other providers. This prompted us to try to obtain a more 'fine-grained' analysis by classifying the soundly evaluated interventions according to key characteristics (type of intervention, age of peer leaders, level of involvement of young people in the development of the intervention etc.) and tabulating them according to the reviewers' judgement about the effectiveness of the intervention (e.g. effective, partly effective, ineffective, harmful, no evidence of effects). However, no clear patterns emerged. We thus had to go back to the individual detail of each study to try to work out why it might be that peer leaders were no more or less effective than other providers. Here we found it invaluable to start to consider the findings from the process evaluations as well. From this, several possible factors emerged, such as the competence of the provider to facilitate learning in groups being the key element rather than the fact that the provider is a 'peer', and the possibility that the greatest effects of the peer education are on the peer educators themselves. Using this synthesis we were able to highlight promising interventions (not necessarily peer-delivered) that needed to be developed and evaluated further. These also included recommending that practitioners should take care to implement peer-delivered health promotion critically, highlighting factors which need to be considered in the implementation of peer-delivered health promotion and recommending that further research needs to be carried out, with practitioners and researchers working in partnership, to understand better what works and what does not work.

The final review 'product'

It is clear from the processes involved at each stage of the review that many different decisions had to be made, all of which had an impact on the final review product. Although we did not consult with all key stakeholder groups (e.g. young people) and did not consult on every decision, we made every effort to engage in a dialogue with potential end-users of the review using existing channels of communication with these users (e.g. peer referee of the proposal for the systematic review and discussion with the steering group). As a result of this dialogue, the final review product involved a mixing of well rehearsed methods in systematic reviewing with new methodological developments. The final report of the review therefore included new sections which mapped the research literature on peer-delivered health promotion and synthesized the findings from process evaluations.

Dissemination of final review products, together with an assessment of their impact, is another area where most work is set in a clinical context (Haines and Donald 1998). Funding usually stops when the review has been completed. We attempted to increase our review's impact by increasing the relevance of its findings to practice. However, we have no formal way of examining whether we achieved this other than through documenting any feedback about the review that we receive or details of how it has been used to influence policy and practice. At the time of writing this chapter, the review has not yet been fully disseminated but we are beginning to receive some positive as well as negative feedback.

For example, peer referees' comments on the draft report indicated that the review would face the resistance to RCTs commonly held within the health promotion field, and raise concerns about practitioners' research being judged by academic standards. More positively, they appreciated the very clear recommendations for policy and practice. They thought that the inclusion of the mapping of research, and process as well as outcome evaluations, added considerable depth and detail to the report; and that the recommendations of the review are likely to have immediate relevance to the field given that there is so much interest from schools and community groups in working with peer education. In terms of its influence on policy and practice, we were informed that policy makers in the Department of Health found the review to be extremely useful in addressing the issue of peer-delivered health promotion for a briefing they had to do for ministers, and the review is currently being used by some members of a specially convened working group organized by the Social Exclusion Unit to explore the relevance of peer education in promoting the health of socially excluded groups.

Of course we cannot definitively conclude that the methodological developments undertaken in this review caused the positive feedback. There may be many other alternative explanations, such as an increase in the use of systematic reviews in general. However, our observations certainly suggest that a timely systematic review conducted on a popular approach to health promotion in a manner relevant to potential users of the review is less likely to meet the fate of so much research: the high dusty bookshelf!

Conclusions

The key messages from this chapter are:

- As systematic reviews attempt to bridge the gap between practice and research, it is essential that they (a) are carried out in a way that assures quality and (b) have findings which are relevant and applicable to the people who need to use them.
- The needs of review users need to be carefully balanced with the need for ensuring that recommendations are based on high-quality evidence and the specific resource constraints of a review.
- Demands for relevance from the systematic review user community force researchers to reflect critically on the methods they use for conducting reviews.
- Systematically engaging in a dialogue with those users, and engendering responsive practice in research, can lead to reviews which are more likely to meet the information needs of policy and practice, and stimulate important methodological developments.

References

Boulton, M., Fitzpatrick, R. and Swinburn, C. (1996) Qualitative research in health care, II: a structured review and evaluation of studies. *Journal of Evaluation in Clinical Practice*, 2(3), 171–9.

Chalmers, I., Enkin, M., and Keirse, M. J. (1989) *Effective Care in Pregnancy and Childbirth*. Oxford: Oxford University Press.

Charleston, S., Oakley, A., Johnson, A. et al. (1996) Report on a Pilot Study for a Randomised Controlled Trial of Peer-led Sex Education in Schools. London: Institute of Education.

Cobb, A. K. and Hagemaster, J. N. (1987) Ten criteria for evaluating qualitative research proposals. Journal of Nursing Education, 26(4), 138–43.

Haines, A. and Donald, A. (eds) (1998) Getting Research Findings into Practice. London: BMJ Publishing Group.

Harden, A., Peersman, G., Oliver, S., Mauthner, M. and Oakley, A. (1999b) A systematic review of the effectiveness of health promotion interventions in the workplace. Occupational Medicine, 49, 1–9.

Harden, A., Weston, R. and Oakley, A. (1999a) A review of the Effectiveness and Appropriateness of Peer-delivered Health Promotion for Young People. London: EPI-Centre, Social Science Research Unit

MacDonald, G., Sheldon, B. and Gillespie, J. (1992) Contemporary studies of the effectiveness of social work. British Journal of Social Work, 22, 615–43.

Mays, N. and Pope, C. (1995) Rigour and qualitative research. British Medical Journal, 311, 109–12.

Medical Sociology Group (1996) Criteria for the evaluation of qualitative research papers. Medical Sociology News, 22(1), 69–71.

Milburn, K. (1995) A critical review of peer education with young people with special reference on sexual health. Health Education Research, 10(4), 407–20.

Oakley, A. (2000) Experiments in Knowing: Gender and Method in the Social Sciences. Cambridge: Polity Press.

Oakley, A., Fullerton, D., Holland, J. et al. (1995) Sexual health education interventions for young people: a methodological review. British Medical Journal, 310, 158–62.

Oliver, S., Milne, R., Bradburn, J. et al. (2001) Involving consumers in a needs-led research programme: a pilot study. Health Expectations, 4(1), 18–28.

Oliver, S., Nicholas, A. and Oakley, A. (1996) Promoting Health after Sifting the Evidence. London: EPI-Centre, Social Science Research Unit.

Peersman, G., Harden, A., Oliver, S. and Oakley, A. (1998) Reviews of Effectiveness in Health Promotion: A Report for the Department of Health. London: EPI-Centre, Social Science Research Unit.

Peersman, G., Oakley, A., Oliver, S. and Thomas, J. (1996) Review of Effectiveness of Sexual Health Promotion Interventions for Young People. London: EPI-Centre, Social Science Research Unit.

Peersman, G. and Oliver, S. (1997) EPI-Centre Keywording Strategy. London: EPI-Centre, Social Science Research Unit.

Peersman, G., Oliver, S. and Oakley, A. (1997) EPI-Centre Review Guidelines. London: EPI-Centre, Social Science Research Unit.

Svenson, G. R. (1998) European Guidelines for Youth AIDS Peer Education. Stockholm: European Commission.

Wilton, T., Keeble, S., Doyal, L., Walsh, A., University of the West of England and South West Regional Health Authority (1995) The Effectiveness of Peer Education in Health Promotion: Theory and Practice. Bristol: University of West England.

▶ 9

▷ Who's listening? Systematically reviewing for ethics and empowerment

▷ Angela Harden and Sandy Oliver

The past quarter-century has seen an important vision emerging within health promotion concerning the people it is designed to serve. No longer is the public seen as the passive recipient of professional intervention, but as an active partner in defining needs and developing solutions for health. The terms 'empowerment', 'participation', 'healthy alliances' and 'partnerships' are qualities to aspire to and frequently feature in discussions about the philosophy and practice of health promotion. Indeed, the concept of empowerment is at the heart of the World Health Organization definition of health promotion as the 'process of enabling people to increase control over, and to improve, their health' (WHO 1986). The importance of empowerment and working in partnership with individuals, communities and organizations is often highlighted in the context of promoting the health of traditionally disadvantaged groups and is at the heart of ethical interventions and research (see Chapter 1).

To what extent this vision is being implemented in practice is, however, a point of contention. Some have argued that it merely represents a change in the language of the 'new' health promotion which masks a continued 'top-down' approach (Robertson and Minkler 1994; Peersman 1998). Although slow to follow, recent UK health policy is now beginning to reflect some of this intended vision. The White Paper *Saving Lives* (Department of Health 1999) proposes a 'national contract for better health', sharing responsibility for a concerted and coordinated drive against poor health between government and national players, local players and communities, and the general public. Throughout, the report makes suggestions for what each of these groups may address together to improve health, but not how.

Taking this vision from 'rhetoric' to 'reality' is likely to be a considerable challenge for those working to promote health, and even more so in research and development, which is often seen as a particularly specialist

activity where new ways of working in partnership can challenge professionals' thinking (Oliver 1999). Building on the issues raised in Chapter 1,
this chapter aims to explore these challenges by examining how ethics and
empowerment feature in health promotion intervention development and
research for a specific group: young people. First, though, the chapter considers in more detail the notion of ethical research.

Ethical research and 'consumer involvement' in research

Ethical research takes account of the aims and effects of research, of the
benefits it might bring and the harms it might inflict. Traditionally, research
ethics have focused on the relationship between researchers and research
participants. The inherent imbalance of this relationship is because of an
unequal access to information and influence in the research process (Hood
et al. 1999). Advances in research ethics are set in the context of increasing
involvement of patients and the public in making decisions about their own
personal health care and about the development and delivery of services.
Pressure for this increasing involvement comes from individual patients
and service users, their families and carers, and organized groups of such
people. Taken together, the activities of these individuals and groups are
recognized as a social movement (Smith and Pillemar 1983). They challenge the professionally dominated social structure indirectly by using and
developing alternative services within the voluntary or commercial sectors
and directly by calling for change in established/statutory services, during
clinical encounters, through complaints procedures and campaigning. Professionals meet these challenges either with resistance or by actively engaging
with the changes (and their agents) that social movements bring.

Members of the public are inevitably involved in health research, even if
only as passive participants, but there is the potential for them to play more
active roles in setting the research agenda, helping to get research funded,
designing and conducting research, reporting and disseminating the findings
and using them to inform policy and practice (Oliver 1999). Advances such
as these are commonly referred to as 'consumer involvement' in research.
Here the term 'consumer' refers to people whose primary interest in health
care is their own health or that of their family, as past, current and potential patients, users of services or carers and people representing any of these
groups through community organizations, networks or campaigning and
self-help groups. The concept of a 'health services consumer' and its associated implications have been critiqued in the sociological literature, especially for their implicit reference to an economic model of supply and
demand. This over-estimates the degree of equality obtaining between
those who provide and those who use health care, and ignores the role of
relatives, friends and neighbours (usually women) as part of an 'informal

economy' in producing and maintaining health (van den Heuvel 1980; Rifkin 1981; Calnan 1988; Stacey 1996).

Consumer involvement in research has emerged from consumer involvement in service planning and is particularly advanced in social care (Nuffield Institutes for Health 1996). Here it is valued as both a political activity and a route to better science (Fisher 1998; Porro 1999). It is sometimes led by consumers (Wiltshire Community Care User Involvement Network 1996; Evans and Fisher 1999), thereby changing the researchers' relationships with 'the researched' and the nature of the 'problem' to be researched (Davis and Fleming 1992).

Consumer activity has roots both in self-help advocacy and in the 'business' approach of agencies in the 1980s, which emphasized listening to customers and being responsive to their needs and preferences. This has been applied directly for the development of wheelchairs and other assistive devices by the use of focus groups and questionnaires with members of consumer networks (Brienza *et al.* 1995). However, such examples are relatively rare.

Researchers who understand that social research can be harmful, and that poor research wastes resources and can misdirect future decisions about health, have responded to this social movement by asking themselves pertinent questions about participants' informed consent and broader ethical issues (Alderson 1995).

Ethical health promotion research: why is it important to listen to young people?

Over the past few decades, young people have been consistently identified as a key group for health promotion interventions both for their vulnerability to adverse health outcomes and for the fact that many health behaviour patterns in later life may be influenced during adolescence (Gillies and McVey 1996). As professionals involved in research, practice or policy-making, we have an ethical duty to make sure that interventions for young people are actually doing the 'good' we think they are doing. Not only is listening to young people an ethical imperative, it has been argued that it is only by taking into account young people's own health needs and agendas that the most effective and appropriate strategies for promoting health will be developed. Health is shaped by specific social, cultural and economic factors and these need to be understood within the specific context of young people's everyday lives (e.g. Aggleton 1992; Wight 1992; Schucksmith and Hendry 1998). This requires us to listen to young people's views about their own health, what they see influencing it and what they would like to see changed. In line with this, there have been calls for the conventional top-down, expert-led models of health promotion to be replaced by active participation of young people in working out ways in which their own health needs can be met (Brannen *et al.* 1994; Peersman 1996). Thus, fundamental to the concept of ethical health promotion research for young people, which informs and empowers, is the notion of 'listening' to them: enabling them to have a voice, hearing what they say and subsequently enabling them and their views to play an active role in shaping any programme design and evaluation.

The rest of this chapter examines the extent to which empowerment and participation feature in recent health promotion research for young people.

Does health promotion research listen to young people?

The overall picture

In order to examine whether ethics and empowerment are features of health promotion for young people, we have drawn on the studies included in two recent systematic reviews conducted at the EPPI-Centre. The first is a systematic review of the effectiveness of sexual health interventions for young people (Peersman *et al.* 1996) and the second the systematic review of the appropriateness and effectiveness of peer-delivered health promotion for young people (Harden *et al.* 1999) discussed in the previous chapter. In total, these reviews included 162 studies which evaluated a health promotion intervention targeted at young people. These studies consisted of outcome evaluations (studies which aimed to examine whether interventions led to a change in health-related outcomes), process evaluations (studies which aimed to examine implementation issues) or studies that included both process and outcome measures. The outcome evaluations employed a range of designs, including randomized controlled trials (RCTs), non-randomized trials and designs which did not include a control or comparison group. The interventions tested focused on a range of health topics, such as the prevention of HIV/AIDS, unintended pregnancy, drug use, smoking and violence. They were implemented in a variety of settings, including community sites, educational institutions and health care settings, with a range of intervention strategies, such as providing information, building skills and modifying the environment.

Detailed data were abstracted from each of the 162 studies using a standardized approach (Peersman *et al.* 1997; see Chapter 7): characteristics of the study population, the type and content of the intervention delivered, planning and process measures and the characteristics and quality of the evaluation. This process allows for the systematic gathering of effectiveness data, as well as data on ethics and empowerment. The relevant questions were:

Did the young people influence the intervention?
• Was the intervention based on a needs assessment?
• Who identified the aims of the intervention?

- Who was involved in the development of the intervention? Did the young people play a role in the evaluation?
- Who carried out the evaluation?
- Were views on the evaluation design sought?
- Who identified the range of processes/outcomes to be addressed?
- To whom were the results of the evaluation reported?

For informed consent

- Was informed consent sought before participants took part in the study?
- If so, from whom (participants, parents or guardians, teachers)?

The planning and development of health promotion programmes for young people

To what extent have young people played a role in the development of health promotion interventions designed for them? Table 9.1 shows the way in which the interventions evaluated in the 162 studies were planned and developed. In particular, it shows whether interventions were based on the needs expressed by young people themselves, whether young people played a part in identifying the aims of the intervention and whether young people played a role in developing the intervention. The proportion of studies which worked in partnership in some way with young people in planning the development of the intervention is very small. Only five (3 per cent) interventions were implemented based on the self-defined needs of

Table 9.1 Number and proportion of studies (N = 162) in reviews of sexual health promotion and peer-delivered health promotion for young people according to the strategies used to plan and develop the interventions which were evaluated

	N	%
Needs assessment		
Driven by 'experts' or other adults (e.g. teachers)	150	93
Needs expressed by young people	5	3
Not stated/unclear	7	4
Identification of aims of the intervention		
Identified by 'experts' or other adults (e.g. teachers)	109	67
Identified in partnership with young people	3	2
Not stated	50	31
Development of intervention		
Developed by 'experts' (e.g. health professionals)	100	62
Developed in partnership with young people	21	13
Not stated	41	25

young people. In three (2 per cent) studies the aims of the intervention were defined in partnership with young people. A slightly larger proportion of studies (21; 13 per cent) evaluated interventions which had been developed in partnership with young people.

All five intervention studies based on self-defined needs were implemented in educational and community settings. Three aimed to promote sexual health (Lamberti and Chapel 1977; McLean 1994; Kegeles *et al.* 1996), one aimed to reduce the onset and amount of alcohol consumption (Perry *et al.* 1993) and one aimed to increase healthy eating and physical activity and prevent smoking in the context of cardiovascular disease (Perry *et al.* 1989). How young people's self-defined needs were elicited varied from study to study. For example, Perry and colleagues (1993) carried out focus groups with young people from the targeted communities to determine what young people saw as the problems facing them related to alcohol; Lamberti and Chapel (1977) simply report that there were unmet demands regarding 'sexual dysfunction' among students at the university where the sexual health intervention was implemented, without expanding on how these demands were expressed.

Of the three studies in which young people played a role in identifying the aims of the intervention, one was an intervention to promote sexual health in an educational setting (Lamberti and Chapel 1977), one aimed to promote safe sex among young gay men implemented in a community setting (Kegeles *et al.* 1996) and one was an intervention aiming to promote safer sex for disadvantaged African American young women (DiClemente and Wingood 1995). Limited information is provided on how the partnerships with young people worked in this respect. Lamberti and Chapel (1977) and DiClemente and Wingood (1995) state that young people were involved in identifying aims; Kegeles *et al.* (1996) indicate that the decisions about the types and aims of the interventions were made by a 'core group' made up of young gay men.

A similarly varied picture is apparent with respect to how young people were engaged in partnerships with professionals in developing interventions. Interestingly, many of these involved 'peer education', which several authors have argued is a method with more potential for creating opportunities for partnership with young people (e.g. Hart 1998; Svenson 1998). Again, the nature of partnerships varied across the 21 studies. For some, the young people's role was confined to one component of the intervention. For example, a video component used in an HIV prevention intervention was performed and written by local teenagers (Quirk *et al.* 1993). Elsewhere, young people designed the content of weekly messages about violence in the context of a wider violence prevention intervention developed by researchers (Orpinas *et al.* 1995). In other studies, young people designed and developed the content of all intervention activities in partnership with health promoter practitioners or researchers (Kegeles *et al.* 1996; Macri and Tsiantis 1997). Though some authors dedicated a separate publication to describing how the interventions were developed (Perry *et al.* 1989), the reporting on these partnerships was often poor. For example, in the outcome evaluation of an intervention to increase safer sex among young African American women, the role of young people in the development of the intervention was described as 'developed by the research team with several young adult African American women from the neighbourhood' (DiClemente and Wingood 1995: 1272).

The evaluation of health promotion programmes for young people

Although there was only a small minority of studies which reported engaging young people in some way in the planning and development of interventions, no studies reported the involvement of young people in the evaluation of interventions. The majority of health promotion interventions were evaluated by researchers alone (92 per cent), with a smaller number being carried out by other professionals, such as health promotion practitioners or health professionals. Similarly, in terms of identifying the range of processes and outcomes to be addressed, none of the studies allowed a role for young people. However, in a few cases (6; 3 per cent) young people were asked for their views on the design of the evaluation. Seeking views, however, was confined to researchers simply testing out data collection instruments for assessing the effectiveness of the intervention (Thomas *et al.* 1985; Hernandez and Smith 1990; Jorgensen 1991; Shulkin *et al.* 1991; Michaud and Hausser 1992; Eisen *et al.* 1992). Only one study reported telling the young people involved the findings of the evaluation (Hauser and Michaud 1994).

Informed consent

Just over half (52 per cent; 82) of all the 162 studies in our sample did not report seeking informed consent from the participants before they took part in the evaluation study: 28 per cent (46) requested consent from the young people themselves and 29 per cent (47) requested consent from others such as parents or legal guardians. Of those studies which sought informed consent (78), 60 per cent (47) stated the numbers consenting, ranging from 20 to 100 per cent (mean 88 per cent). Such a wide range reflects not only on how people view the research but also on how consent is sought. Consent may be 'required', or only 'implied' if young people or those acting on their behalf are informed about the research study and choose not to exclude themselves. In the trial of sex education described in Chapter 10, the ethics committee insisted that parental consent be sought for the sex education programme.

Partnership in practice

One study stands out for combining sound design for assessing effectiveness with a participative philosophy in developing and delivering the intervention. Kegeles *et al.* (1996) evaluated a peer-led community-based HIV prevention intervention for young men who have sex with men. The aim of the intervention was to mobilize and empower the young gay men's community to encourage and support each other about the need for safer sex. As many young men as possible were recruited as 'peer leaders', and each one was considered a potential agent for change. These peer leaders were central to the development, content and delivery of the intervention. Four young gay men were employed part-time as project coordinators and a core group of 12 to 15 young gay men served as the decision-making body for the project. For instance, they designed outreach materials and procedures, and a wider team of young gay men undertook the outreach work. These procedures were incorporated within the context of an RCT set in two Californian cities.

Working in partnership is not always easy, and some research teams investigated this aspect with young people. The Fife Healthcare NHS Trust (1996) evaluation found major problems with coordinators supporting programmes and peer leaders. While one coordinator expected and accommodated the personal development of the peer educators during the course of the programme, other coordinators found it difficult when the young peer educators began to express their own ideas, needs and wants. Similarly, Peers *et al.* (1993) found working with young people to be challenging. In particular, such partnerships were not always felt to lead to the best use of resources, and working partnerships had to be reassessed in order to provide the necessary organization, discipline and control, while ensuring the peer educators felt a sense of ownership of the project. This is documented in the literature on student-centred participative approaches to learning (see, for example, Weston 1986). However much they believe in equity and partnerships, professionals tend to seek to retake control when things do not go as planned. To some extent problems are inevitable in projects which encourage young people to take the initiative, yet are still bound by the constraints of school or college environments (Fife Healthcare NHS Trust 1996: 43). Massey and Neidigh (1990) illustrated how autonomy can be returned to young people. In their evaluation of a peer-based alcohol programme in a university setting, the power differential between peer educators and professionals was realigned by taking a step back to evaluate the problems. Following this, explicit decision-making procedures were set out. Although initially the young people needed support for making decisions, they gradually adapted to their position of control and responsibility.

Considering the difficulties encountered when young people work as 'equal partners' with professionals in developing and delivering interventions, it is not surprising that young people's active involvement in the more complex task of evaluating these interventions was virtually non-existent. This is not to say that young people never influence research or evaluation or, indeed, take the lead, but such examples are rare, not only in health promotion but in health research generally.

Why doesn't health promotion research listen to young people?

The analysis presented in this chapter does not give a very encouraging picture in terms of health promotion research listening to young people. The majority of interventions evaluated in the studies included in this analysis were implemented on the basis of expert opinion, with few involving young people in their development. Many interventions were reported to be developed on the basis of a theoretical model. This may well be important for helping to base the intervention content on the theoretical determinants of health and health behaviours (e.g. enhancing self-efficacy, teaching skills to resist social pressure) or style of delivery (e.g. didactic versus interactive presentation). However, as several authors note, an over-reliance on theory, especially individualistic psychological theory, can actually serve to neglect the needs and views of the target population (Bunton et al. 1991), unless the theory is grounded in their experiences in the first place. Even when reports described interventions as aiming to empower or work in partnership with young people, many of these showed a significant gap between what they said they were aiming to do and what actually happened in practice. In particular, the reluctance of adults to devolve power to young people, and institutional structures demarcating appropriate adult and child roles, made it difficult for the principles of empowerment to be put into practice.

To some extent, the difficulties in working in equal partnerships with young people reflect the implications of the way this population group is socially and culturally constructed, characterized by its 'non-adult' status (Mayall 1994; Moore and Kindness 1998). Academic and everyday views of 'children' and 'young people' portray them as innocent, vulnerable and in need of protection, naughty and in need of discipline and guidance, or as second class citizens less important than adults. They are often treated as a homogeneous group, ignoring important differences in their experiences according to, for example, class and gender. These constructions have had two major consequences: we currently know very little about the views and experiences of young people, and little importance is given to how young people understand their role and actions in the social world (Moore and Kindness 1998). For health promotion, this means that, despite good intentions, interventions are primarily driven by an 'adult' agenda, which defines what problems need to be tackled and how (Milburn 1995; Shucksmith and Hendry 1998). Two topical issues illustrate how 'problems' and 'solutions' can be turned upside down when the adult or professional agenda is not prioritized. The perennial problem of school bullying has traditionally been seen as a discipline issue, where the authority (and power) of teachers is to be enforced. More recently it has been recognized specifically as a human rights issue, with the right to protection from violence being enshrined in the UN Convention on the rights of the child (Lansdown 1999). A less common experience is that of young people caring for sick or disabled parents. The problem of 'young carers' has attracted the attention of the authorities, who have considered it in terms of interference with young people's school work and social life. Seen from the families' point of view, however, the primary problem is the lack of support for the sick or disabled parent.

A recent expert working group on promoting the health of children and young people has begun some work on this issue, recommending a new research agenda that takes into account the social construction of childhood and young people. This agenda specifically calls for a re-evaluation of participatory approaches with young people (HEA 1998).

While work in partnership with young people to promote their health may appear limited, these limitations are seen across the age range (see Harden et al. 1999 for workplace health promotion, and Chapter 6 for promoting the health of older people), in health services other than health promotion and across health services research generally.

Successful partnerships

Health promotion has a creditable record for establishing working partnerships, albeit often restricted to the stage of need assessment. A case study of 15 partnerships in health promotion between the NHS and voluntary organizations identified common factors which were thought to enhance their success: the influence of a 'mentor' figure at a senior level within the Health Service or the Department of Health; flexible, dynamic project leadership retaining key staff; skills and credibility within the voluntary sector partners; mutual respect and understanding; a businesslike approach, with voluntary organizations enabled to contribute rather than swamped with tasks they cannot manage; evaluation; and funding (Fieldgrass 1992). This represents considerable investment of effort and resources by authorities in empowering others to work with them. Although this effort can be made and prove fruitful in research contexts too (Oliver 1995, 1999), it is unusual.

Chapter 10 provides a practical example of how young people can be consulted throughout the research process, and contribute constructively to the development of both the methods of and the intervention tested in an RCT of school-based peer-delivered sex education.

Conclusions

There are strong arguments for engaging young people as partners in the development of health promotion. Only some health promotion interventions for young people are implemented on the basis of a thorough assessment of both young people's self-defined health needs and their views on what kind of intervention they would find most appropriate, taking into account young people's values and the social and material context of their lives.

For several reasons, professionals may find it difficult to work in equal partnerships with young people. Resource constraints may be a very real barrier and conflicting value systems concerning young people's autonomy may be a particular problem when working within school-based contexts. There are, however, lessons to be learned from the existing literature. Recognition of young people as a heterogeneous group calls for research for and with different subgroups of young people. The boundaries of working in partnership with young people need to be established in consultation with all stakeholders prior to project implementation. As young people are rarely, if ever, actively involved in prioritizing, developing and soundly evaluating the effects of interventions, we can only speculate about the material benefits of this approach.

The key messages from this chapter are:

- Advances in research ethics have been made in the context of increasing involvement of the public in making decisions about their own personal health and about the development and delivery of services.
- Despite these advances, young people are often overlooked when informed consent is sought in health promotion research.
- Health promotion and the notion of ethical research embody the principles of listening to, and working in partnership with, the individuals and groups they are intended to serve.
- An increase in calls for partnership within the discursive health promotion literature is not matched by partnerships in practice with young people involved in developing and evaluating interventions.
- Effort needs to be invested in overcoming the barriers to engaging young people in designing and evaluating health promotion interventions for them.

References

Aggleton, P. (ed.) (1992) *Young People and HIV/AIDS*. Papers from an ESRC-sponsored seminar on young people and HIV/AIDS social research. London: ESRC/Health and Education Research Unit, University of London.

Alderson, P. (1995) *Listening to Children: Children, Ethics and Social Research*. London: Barnardo's.

Brannen, J., Dodd, K., Oakley, A. and Storey, P. (1994) *Young People, Health and Family Life*. Buckingham: Open University Press.

Brienza, D., Angelo, J. and Henry, K. (1995) Consumer participation in identifying research and development priorities for power wheelchair input devices and controllers. *Assistive-Technology*, 7(1), 55–62.

Bunton, R., Murphy, S. and Bennett, P. (1991) Theories of behavioural change and their use in health promotion: some neglected areas. *Health Education Research*, 6, 153–62.

Calnan, M. (1988) Towards a conceptual framework of lay evaluation in health care. *Social Science and Medicine*, 27(9), 927–33.

Davis, A. and Fleming, A. (1992) User-commissioned research – the shape of things to come? *Social Services Research Source Info*, 1, 50–3.

Department of Health (1999) *Saving Lives: Our Healthier Nation*. London: HMSO.

DiClemente, R. J. and Wingood, G. M. (1995) A randomized controlled trial of an HIV sexual risk-reduction intervention for young African-American women. *Journal of the American Medical Association*, 274(16), 1271–6.

Eisen, M., Zellman, G. L. and McAlister, A. L. (1992) A health belief model–social learning theory approach to adolescents' fertility control: findings from a controlled field trial. *Health Education Quarterly*, 19(2), 249–62.

Evans, C. and Fisher, M. (1999) Collaborative evaluation with service users: moving towards user-controlled research. In I. Shaw and J. Lishman (eds) *Evaluation and Social Work Practice*. London: Sage.

Fieldgrass, J. (1992) *Partnerships in Health Promotion: Collaboration between the Statutory and Voluntary Sectors*. London: Health Education Authority and National Council for Voluntary Organisations.

Fife Healthcare NHS Trust (1996) *Peer Education HIV/AIDS Evaluation Report, 1,2 and 3*. Fife: Fife Healthcare NHS Trust.

Fisher, M. (1998) The role of service users in problem formation and technical aspects of social research. Paper presented at a conference on user involvement organized by SPRU, York University.

Gillies, P. and McVey, D. (1996) *Research for Health Promotion. A Research Strategy for the Health Education Authority for England 1996–1999*. London: Health Education Authority.

Harden, A., Weston, R. and Oakley, A. (1999) *A Systematic Review of the Effectiveness and Appropriateness of Health Promotion Interventions for Young People*. London: EPI-Centre, Social Science Research Unit.

Hart, G. J. (1998) Peer education and community based HIV prevention for homosexual men: peer led, evidence based, or fashion driven? *Sexually Transmitted Infections*, 74, 87–94.

Hausser, D. and Michaud, P. A. (1994) Does a condom-promoting strategy (the swiss-stop-AIDS-campaign) modify sexual-behavior among adolescents. *Pediatrics*, 93(4), 580–5.

Health Education Authority (1998) *Promoting the Health of Children and Young People: Setting a Research Agenda*. London: Health Education Authority.

Hernandez, J. T. and Smith, F. J. (1990) Abstinence, protection, and decision-making: experimental trials on prototypic AIDS programs. *Health Education Research*, 5(3), 309–20.

Hood, S., Mayall, B. and Oliver, S. (1999) *Critical Issues in Social Research: Power and Prejudice*. Buckingham: Open University Press.

Jorgensen, S. R. (1991) Project taking charge: an evaluation of an adolescent pregnancy prevention program. *Family Relations*, 40, 373–80.

Kegeles, S. M., Hays, R. B. and Coates, T. J. (1996) The Mpowerment project: a community-level HIV prevention intervention for young gay men. *American Journal of Public Health*, 86(81), 1129–36.

Lamberti, J. and Chapel, J. (1977) Development and evaluation of a sex education program for medical students. *Journal of Medical Education*, 52, 582–5.

Lansdown, G. (1999) The UN Convention on the Rights of the Child: implications for education. Paper presented to the Summerhill conference on the free child, July.

McLean, D. A. (1994) A model for HIV risk reduction and prevention among African American college students. *Journal of American College Health*, 42(5), 220–3.

Macri, I. and Tsiantis, J. (1997) Effects of a peer led intervention program on smoking prevention: a case example in Greece. *International Quarterly of Community Health Education*, 17, 297–308.

Massey, R. F. and Neidigh, L. W. (1990) Evaluating and improving the functioning of a peer-based alcohol abuse prevention organisation. *Journal of Alcohol and Drug Education*, 35(2), 24–35.

Mayall, B. (1994) *Children, Health and the Social Order*. Buckingham: Open University Press.

Michaud, P. A. and Hausser, D. (1992) Swiss teenagers, AIDS and sexually transmitted diseases: presentation and evaluation of a preventive exhibition. *Health Education Research*, 7(1), 79–82.

Milburn, K. (1995) A critical review of peer education with young people with special reference on sexual health. *Health Education Research*, 10(4), 407–20.

Moore, H. and Kindness, L. (1998) Establishing a research agenda for the health and wellbeing of children and young people in the context of health promotion. In Health Education Authority (eds) *Promoting the Health of Children and Young People: Setting a Research Agenda*. London: Health Education Authority.

Nuffield Institute for Health (1996) *User Involvement in Research. The Collaborative Centre for Priority Services Research, Bulletin No. 3*. Leeds: Nuffield Institute for Health.

Oliver, S. (1995) How can health service users contribute to the NHS research and development programme? *British Medical Journal*, 310, 1318–20.

Oliver, S. (1999) Users of health services: following their agenda. In S. Hood, B. Mayall and S. Oliver (eds) *Critical Issues in Social Research: Power and Prejudice*. Buckingham: Open University Press.

Orpinas, P., Parcel, G. S., McAlister, A. and Frankowski, R. (1995) Violence prevention in middle schools: a pilot evaluation. *Journal of Adolescent Health*, 17, 360–71.

Peers, I. S., Leadwith, F. and Johnston, M. (1993) *Community Youth Project on HIV/AIDS: Draft Final Report to Health Education Authority*. Manchester: University of Manchester.

Peersman, G. (1996) *A Descriptive Mapping of Health Promotion Studies in Young People*. London: EPI-Centre, Social Science Research Unit.

Peersman, G. (1998) The 'targets' of health promotion. In S. Hood, B. Mayall and S. Oliver (eds) *Critical Issues in Social Research: Power and Prejudice*. Buckingham: Open University Press.

Peersman, G., Oakley, A., Oliver, S. and Thomas, J. (1996) *Review of Effectiveness of Sexual Health Promotion Interventions for Young People*. London: EPI-Centre, Social Science Research Unit.

Peersman, G., Oliver, S. and Oakley, A. (1997) *EPI-Centre Review Guidelines*. London: EPI-Centre, Social Science Research Unit.

Perry, C. L., Klepp, K. and Sillers, C. (1989) Community wide strategies for cardiovascular health: the Minnesota heart health youth program, *Health Education Research*, 4(1), 87–101.

Perry, C., Williams, C. L., Forster, J. *et al.* (1993) Background, conceptualization and design of a community wide research program on adolescent alcohol use: Project Northland, *Health Education Research*, 8(1), 125–36.

Porro, G. S. (1999) How carers can improve research. Paper presented by the President of Federazione Alzheimer Italia at a meeting of minds – care and science in dementia, Ninth Alzheimer Europe Meeting and Alzheimer's Disease Society Conference, 30 June to 2 July, London.

Quirk, M., Godkin, M. and Schwenzfeier, E. (1993) Evaluation of two AIDS prevention interventions for inner-city adolescent and young adult women. *American Journal of Preventive Medicine*, 9(1), 21–6.

Rifkin, S. B. (1981) The role of the public in planning, management and evaluation of health activities and programmes, including self-care. *Social Science and Medicine*, 15A, 377–86.

Robertson, A. and Minkler, M. (1994) New health promotion movement: a critical examination. *Health Education Quarterly*, 21, 295–312.

Shucksmith, J. and Hendry, L. (1998) *Health Issues and Adolescents: Growing Up, Speaking Out*. London: Routledge.

Shulkin, J. J., Mayer, J. A., Wessel, L. G. *et al.* (1991) Effects of a peer-led AIDS intervention with university students. *Journal of American College Health*, 40 (Sept.), 75–9.

Smith, D. H. and Pillemar, K. (1983) Self help groups as social movement organizations: social structure and social change. *Research in Social Movements, Conflicts and Change*, 5, 203–33.

Stacey, M. (1996) The health service consumer: a sociological misconception. In M. Stacey (ed.) *The Sociology of the NHS*, Sociological Review Monograph 22. Keele: University of Keele.

Svenson, G. R. (1998) *European Guidelines for Youth AIDS Peer Education*. Stockholm: European Commission.

Thomas, L. L., Long, S. E., Whitten, K. *et al.* (1985) High school students' long term retention of sex education information. *Journal of School Health*, 55(7), 274–8.

van den Heuvel, W. J. (1980) The role of the consumer in health policy. *Social Science and Medicine*, 14A: 423–26.

Weston, R. (1986) Self concept and its relationship with life and health choices. Unpublished MA(Ed), University of Southampton.

Wiltshire Community Care User Involvement Network (1996) '*I Am in Control': Research into Users' Views of the Wiltshire Independent Living Fund*. Devizes: Wiltshire and Swindon Users' Network and WCCUIN.

Wight, D. (1992) Impediments to safer heterosexual sex: a review of research with young people. *AIDS Care*, 4(1), 11–22.
World Health Organization (1986). *Ottawa Charter for Health Promotion: an International Conference on Health Promotion.* Copenhagen: WHO Regional Office for Europe.

▷ A listening trial: 'qualitative' methods
within experimental research

▷ **Vicki Strange, Simon Forrest, Ann Oakley
and the RIPPLE Study Team**

Introduction

Literature on health promotion evaluation has emphasized the value of
applying methodological approaches that 'listen' to people and prioritize
the perspectives of research participants (see Chapter 9). Such approaches
are cited in some circles as likely to produce 'better' data and result in
a more ethical research process (Green and Kreuter 1991; Davies and
Macdonald 1998; Moore and Kindness 1998; Weston 1998). At the same
time, experimental methods are increasingly being considered as appropriate and necessary for evaluating social interventions (Oakley and Fullerton
1996; Stephenson and Imrie 1998; Oakley 2000). But these methods are
also often criticized for their lack of focus on participants' perspectives: for
example, when 'objective' outcome data are prioritized over participants'
self-reports of events (Scott 1992; Hunter 1993; Williams and Popay 1997).
The perception that experimental designs are incompatible with respect for
participants' viewpoints may sometimes lead to the conclusion that other
approaches to evaluation need to be used instead.

This chapter describes the way we have sought to integrate complementary research methods in the RIPPLE study. RIPPLE stands for Randomized Intervention of Pupil-Peer Led sex Education; the design is that
of a randomized controlled trial (RCT) evaluating the effectiveness of peer-
led sex education in English secondary schools. The study started in 1997
and will continue, in its present phase of funding, until 2002, so there are
no 'findings' available yet. This chapter illustrates some of the ways in
which an experimental study can incorporate 'people-centred', 'listening'
approaches. First, we briefly describe the rationale for the trial and outline

its design. We next discuss some of the methods being used in the study to obtain 'qualitative' data capable of highlighting the views and perspectives of trial participants, and the advantages and difficulties of using these methods. Our aim is that the chapter will provide readers with ideas about how to integrate 'qualitative' and experimental methods, and with some solutions to possible problems.

Why undertake an RCT and why peer-led sex education?

In the UK, sexual health promotion has become an increasing focus of government policy, with established targets for reducing unintended teenage pregnancy and sexually transmitted diseases (STDs) (DoH 1992). A systematic review in 1995 of sexual health education interventions for young people found that most interventions had not been evaluated, or had been evaluated in such a way that no reliable conclusions about effectiveness could be drawn (Oakley *et al.* 1995). The review recommended the use of well designed RCTs with 5–10 years of follow-up where possible. In July 1999 the Social Exclusion Unit report on teenage pregnancy identified peer-led sex education as a possible prevention strategy. Peer-led approaches are increasingly fashionable. They are recommended in many quarters, both within and outside school settings and for young people as well as other population groups, with much enthusiasm but without much in the way of a firm evidence base (Fennell 1993; Mathie and Ford 1994).

A feasibility study for the RIPPLE project was carried out in four schools in 1996–7, funded by the UK Department of Health. The aim was to address initial questions such as whether it was possible to randomize schools to a control or intervention group, how a complex intervention might best be carried out and which evaluation methods would be most appropriate in the school context (Stephenson *et al.* 1998). The feasibility study found that students in the two schools receiving peer-led sex education positively evaluated the intervention; the study also collected information enabling the further development of the peer-led programme, established that an RCT design in school settings was indeed feasible and initiated work on many of the methods to be used in a larger study.

The feasibility study was carried out by a multidisciplinary team of social and medical scientists at University College and the Institute of Education in London. The same team was funded by the Medical Research Council (MRC) in 1997 to undertake a multisite RCT. A year earlier the MRC had also funded an RCT of teacher-led sex education in Scotland known as SHARE (Sexual Health and Relationships – Safe Happy and Responsible). Both studies are the first of their kind; both are large-scale and long-term, and afford an exciting opportunity to answer many unanswered questions about the short- and long-term effectiveness of sex education in the UK.

The Scottish and English research teams are collaborating to use some of the same methods and measures, so the results of the two trials can be compared. The questionnaires used in the RIPPLE trial also incorporate questions used in the National Survey of Sexual Attitudes and Lifestyles (Johnson *et al.* 1994).

The RIPPLE intervention and design

In 1997, 27 schools were recruited across England and randomly allocated either to receive the peer-led intervention or to act as control schools. The control schools received some money which they could use on anything except on providing enhanced sex education; hence, they continued with their usual sex education curriculum.

The peer-led intervention was developed by an external team of experienced practitioners in the field of sexual health promotion. Volunteers were recruited from year 12 students (aged 16–17) and took part in a brief training course which provided them with information relating to sexual health issues and teaching/presentation methods. These volunteers, in groups of two to four, then led sex education sessions with two successive cohorts of year 9 students (aged 13–14). They delivered three one-hour sessions covering the topics of relationships, STDs and contraception.

The main method of data collection in the RIPPLE trial to date is self-administered questionnaires completed by approximately 4,500 students in each cohort during classroom time. Baseline and post-intervention information (initially after six months and two years) is gathered from year 9 students, including measures of knowledge, attitudes and behaviour. The questionnaires were developed in consultation with students, and use an accessible and attractive layout with space for comments. Where possible someone from the research team is present to explain the aims of the research, reassure students of the confidentiality of their responses and answer any queries. The trial is currently in its third year and a second (2 year) follow-up has been completed with the first cohort of (now) year 11 students. The two-year follow-up will be carried out with the second cohort in spring 2001. Longer-term follow-up to the age of 18 is also planned, when outcomes will include measures of STDs and pregnancy rates.

An extensive process evaluation is an integral part of the research design. The primary aims of this are: to document how the intervention is implemented in the experimental schools, and what kind of sex education is provided in control schools; to collect information from all the study schools about the experience and impact of taking part in the RIPPLE study; to examine the extent to which sex education in control schools may have been 'contaminated' by knowledge about the peer-led programme; and to collect data on the key processes involved in the provision and receipt of peer-led

sex education, which can then help to interpret 'outcome' data. Information is being gathered about all key events in the peer-led intervention across all experimental schools and sex education lessons in a sample of control schools. In addition, we are trying to gain as much information as possible about the school environments in which the trial is taking place.

Some process information is gathered when students complete the questionnaires. However, most of it is obtained by using other methods, including focus groups, interviews with students and staff and observations of training and delivery sessions. These methods potentially give access to the perspectives of all those involved. Because of the possible influence of the research activities themselves (the so-called 'Hawthorne' effect), observations and focus groups are being carried out in half of the control schools only. The aim here is to compare these schools with those omitted from the process evaluation, so that the effect of the research activities on processes and outcomes can be assessed. Figure 10.1 shows the different research activities involving both year 9 and year 12 students up to the end of 1999 and their timing in relation to the intervention.

Process and outcome evaluations should not be assumed to be associated with 'qualitative' and 'quantitative' methods or data respectively. For example, 'qualitative' methods such as interviews can provide 'quantitative' data which can be used to assess outcome. It would also be misleading to assume that 'qualitative' methods are necessarily more people-centred and participative; involving research participants fully in the research process as informed, consenting individuals is a challenge and a possibility irrespective of the research method being used (Oakley 1998a).

The RIPPLE study involves a complex intervention and a multiplicity of methods and data. The following sections concentrate on only a subset of these; they illustrate how four methods of collecting 'qualitative' data – focus groups, observations, researcher fieldnotes and comments written in questionnaires – are being used in the study to access the views and perspectives of the young people taking part in it.

Description of some methods used to collect qualitative data

Focus groups

Much has been written about the advantages of using focus groups to access participants' views, and on the issues that should be considered when recruiting participants and facilitating groups (see, for example, Basch 1987; Kitzinger 1995). The aim of using focus groups in the RIPPLE study is to gain insight into students' perceptions and evaluation of sex education: what they liked and disliked, why they thought parts of the sessions were

Figure 10.1   Timing of research activities in relation to the intervention

Research activities		Intervention	
		Experimental schools	Control schools
Autumn 1997	• **Baseline questionnaire to year 9**		
Spring 1998	• Observation of recruitment • Baseline questionnaire with all peer educators • **Interviews with teachers**	Recruitment of peer educators	Continue with sex education as planned
Summer 1998	• Observation of pre-training and training sessions • **Observation of sex education sessions delivered to year 9*** • Follow-up questionnaire with all peer educators • **Focus groups with year 9 students** • Focus groups with peer educators	Preparatory sessions with peer educators Needs assessment by peer educators with year 9. Training of peer educators. Delivery of sex education classes	Continue with sex education as planned
Autumn 1998	• **Baseline questionnaire to year 9** • **Follow-up questionnaire to year 10**		
Spring 1999	Repeat all of above for cohort 2		
Summer 1999			
Autumn 1999	• **Second follow-up questionnaire to year 11** • **Follow-up questionnaire to year 10**		

Note: All activities in bold were carried out in both experimental and control schools. Others were carried out only in experimental schools.
* Sex education in control schools was observed throughout the year and depended on the timing of delivery which was decided by individual schools.

successful or not, how they perceived the peer educators or teachers as providers of sex education and their views on wider issues about the school environment and culture. By using focus groups as opposed to individual interviews we hoped to (a) be able to access views from more students involved in the study in the time available, (b) provide a less exposing/intimidating context than individual interviews for students to give their views and (c) gain access to additional data regarding students' interaction in general that might point to relevant issues regarding group/class interaction (e.g. differing modes of communication between students of different status).

A number of sometimes conflicting issues had to be considered. Did we want as broad a range of views as possible or access to particularly 'normal' or 'extreme' views? Was it better to have a heterogeneous or homogeneous group? How compatible did the participants need to be for them to feel comfortable, and how might this influence the breadth of the data? Was it better to ask for volunteers, select participants at random or pick particular 'types' of people – and which 'types'?

All these issues involved balancing the feasible with the desirable. Even with decisions made about the 'type' of data, the most appropriate strategy was not always clear. For example, in the interest of generalizability it might have been beneficial to create focus groups consisting of a representative sample of year 9 students. In practice, it was difficult to decide which characteristics (gender, ability, sexual experience?) should be used for sampling, and heterogeneous groups of students would not necessarily feel comfortable with one another. In the end, the focus groups were mainly single-sex groups of students (mixed sex for year 12) who either volunteered to take part or were chosen by teachers with the aim of selecting a 'mix' of people who would feel comfortable talking about sex education. A semi-structured interview schedule was put together and all group sessions were tape recorded.

Observation

In deciding whether or how to use observational methods we had to reflect on their potential advantages and disadvantages. There was some initial concern among the research team that the presence of a researcher during sex education sessions might significantly alter the dynamics, particularly in the peer-led sessions. However, it was clear that no other method could provide detailed data on significant issues such as the way in which peers or teachers delivered the sessions and interacted with the year 9 students, students' responses and the type of language used, and how the peer-led intervention was implemented. Being able to say something reliable about how the intervention of peer-led sex education compared with sex-education-as-normal is a key issue. Many of the advantages cited for peer-led health promotion centre on the increased similarity and shared cultural references/language between pupil deliverers and recipients compared to those existing between teachers and students. Hence, it was extremely important to use a method that would enable some conclusions to be drawn about whether this happens in practice or not, as evidence suggests that the content of school sex education is very variable and overall poorly researched (Pearson 1999; Lawrence et al. 2000).

The extensive literature on participant observation (Spradley 1980; Stenhouse 1982; Burgess 1983; Robson 1993) provided pointers to issues to be considered when deciding how the observations should be carried out. Critical issues were: how structured the observations should be; the role of the observer as active participant or not; what to tell students about the purpose of the observations; how to record, write up and analyse observations; and how to decide who to observe. It was decided to observe the key processes of the intervention in all the experimental schools. This involved observation of meetings with peer volunteers, all training days for the peer volunteers and the same class of year 9 students taking part in three different sex education sessions (usually delivered by same set of peer leaders) in each experimental school. We hoped that by observing the same group of year 9 students for all three sessions we would be able to comment on the development in the relationships between peer volunteers and year 9 students. The disadvantage was that it would be harder to comment on the variability between groups. We also aimed to observe sex education in half of the control schools; no specific criteria were used to select which year 9 classes would be observed. For all the observation sessions, we took a non-participative role which consisted of writing notes from a discrete position in the classroom and avoiding any active interaction. At each event, a full description (narrative) was written, including what was said, who was present, the activities undertaken, interactions between participants, atmosphere and significant events occurring.

The methods used for observation and focus groups were designed and then continually refined through discussions in which the three fieldworkers involved compared their experiences.

Comments on questionnaires

The baseline and follow-up questionnaires included a 'comments box', a space where students were encouraged to write any views they have about sex education, the questionnaire, other aspects of the research procedure or anything else that they felt might be of interest to the research team.

Researcher fieldnotes

Systematic researcher fieldnotes were taken, using a procedure developed in the SHARE trial, in which information relating to the atmosphere and events occurring during the questionnaire administration was recorded. Data on these 'researcher perception sheets' included: students' privacy and the time available for completion of the questionnaire; teachers' presence or not; seating arrangements; and comments made or questions asked by students.

The researchers also collected information relating to the context in which focus groups and observations were carried out (e.g. how students came to take part, where the groups are held, how students/researchers feel about them, how they/we think their views might differ from those of others in the study) and additional information relating to casual conversations and incidents observed throughout the course of conducting research within schools. Gathering these comments and notes provides insight into (a) student responses to particular methods, (b) the way in which the research methods themselves might influence the type of data gathered and (c) the generalizability of the data obtained.

Confidentiality

In order to obtain honest and complete responses, students were assured that all responses (whatever the method of data collection) were confidential. Analysis of students' comments on the questionnaires, and researcher field-notes taken when the questionnaires were being administered, showed this to be an important issue. Although confidentiality was explained and emphasized before the questionnaires were handed out, it was clear that this was an area that needed further attention. For example, comments indicated that a question asking for the students' postcodes (to establish whether they lived near health services) was disliked by many students and so this was removed. Another difficult issue was finding an acceptable way of being able to link baseline and follow-up questionnaires without compromising the confidentiality of students responses. A list of the pupils' names was obtained before we visited the school and each student was allocated a unique numerical code which was then printed on the back of the questionnaire. In the classroom questionnaires had to be given out, ensuring that each student received the correctly coded questionnaire. These lists were not available to anyone outside of the research team. Concern from students that their responses would be traced back to them meant that researchers had to put a considerable amount of effort into improving our explanations of this aspect of the research process as well as making it very clear that if they felt unsure about the confidentiality they could leave out responses to any questions they chose. Students' comments on issues around confidentiality enabled us to adapt our methods and, we hope, improve the quality of the data obtained, while at the same time retaining the principle of confidentiality.

Why are we doing this and what's it got to do with me?
Engagement and understanding the aims of the research

Getting complete data from research participants is contingent on their feeling that the research is worthwhile. A central concern for the research team was ensuring that as many students as possible were engaged by the research. The aims of the research were clearly explained to all students before they took part in any of the research activities. Again comments in the baseline questionnaire assisted in identifying which aspects of the research required clearer explanation. Some of these comments related to the point of the research as a whole: for example, 'why are we doing this?' and (a commonly asked question) 'what are you going to do with all this?' Other comments suggested that some students were concerned or irritated by particular questions and perhaps viewed these as unnecessary, irrelevant or invasive. Some of these were questions relating to social background: for example, 'I believe Q42 (To which of the following groups do you consider you belong?) was a bit racist, that's why I didn't answer' and 'It doesn't matter really what my mum and dad do, it's to do with them and nobody else especially how old my mum is.' Although providing explanations for why these questions were included in the questionnaire may have persuaded some students of their value, it was impossible in the time allowed in most lessons to provide as part of every introduction a rationale for individual questions. Interestingly, the questions relating to students' own sexual activity, which might have been anticipated to cause the greatest concern, were rarely referred to directly in students' comments. This may have been because they could easily understand why these questions had been included in a questionnaire about sexual health.

As well as having a clear understanding of the aims of the research, it is important for participants to have a clear idea of the role and agenda of the researcher. Common questions to the researchers were: 'Are you a teacher?' 'Where are you from?' 'What are you going to do with all this?' (asked, for example, of tape recordings of focus groups). It was felt that being clear about these issues allowed the students to make decisions about what they were willing/able to contribute and in most cases made it possible for them to take a more constructive part in the research.

Whose perspective do we hear?

In applying our methods we were concerned that that they should reflect the diversity of views held by the young people involved in the study. Through examining students' comments in the questionnaires and through researcher fieldnotes we identified a number of ways in which our methods could be improved. For example, fieldnotes referring to sessions during which year 9 students completed questionnaires indicated that some parts of the questionnaire were not easily read or comprehended, particularly by students with a low reading ability. Some examples of the words which caused difficulty were 'failure', 'pregnancy' and 'contraception'. Where possible we assisted students with reading and comprehension, and by asking teachers where to anticipate problems, we were able to focus our resources where they could be of most use. In some classes, a support teacher was also present. In general, students did not seem concerned if their responses were seen by support teachers, and were not embarrassed by asking for help. Some support teachers described their relationships with students as being more informal than students' relationships with other teachers, and cited examples of students choosing to tell them about personal issues that they would not tell teachers. Not all students had the opportunity to seek help from either a researcher or a support teacher, and some may not have wished to ask for help. In some cases questions were left out or inaccurately answered, or questionnaires were not completed.

Fieldnotes and written comments from students indicated that some questions held little or no meaning for them. For example, perceptions of ethnicity or family composition were difficult to capture with closed questions. One question asked both boys and girls about their perceived ability to refuse sex. Some boys were unable to understand why they would want to refuse sex, and so were unable to answer the question. Other comments suggested that some students felt there were aspects of their experiences or issues that they felt were important but on which the questionnaire did not allow them to comment: for example, 'I think that on some of the questions you should be allowed to write what you feel', and 'The questionnaire was OK but you did not ask many questions on love and feelings, e.g. have you thought you have been in love? Or how did it end, how did it feel? It would have made the questionnaire more enjoyable (well for me) and I think that it related (relates) to sex in more ways than one.'

Reading these comments helped us to identify areas of young people's experience that could be included in follow-up questionnaires and/or explored further through focus groups. It could be argued that most of the issues noted in relation to young people's experiences with completing the RIPPLE questionnaires should have been picked up in the feasibility study. But although the questionnaires were based on those piloted in the feasibility study, it is always difficult to anticipate the range of responses likely to be elicited in other, larger samples.

The way in which students were recruited to take part in focus groups had implications for the extent to which the data reflect a diversity of views. In most schools teachers were asked to select students they felt would feel comfortable talking about their sex education. This may have resulted in particular types of students, perhaps those considered confident and/or those well liked by teachers, being given the opportunity to express their views. Sometimes we were able to ask for volunteers from the whole class; but it seemed that in front of other students only certain people felt able or willing to volunteer, again either the people who were most engaged with the lesson or those who were most dominant within the group and whose views had been most visible throughout the lesson. In one case (in a control school where teacher sex education had been observed), no girls volunteered for the focus group. After the lesson, the class teacher explained that the boys within this group were very dominating and he suggested that the researcher should take all the girls to a separate room and talk to them as a whole group about their experiences. Concerned that the girls were being pushed to take part in something they did not want to, the researcher decided simply to ask the girls why they had not wanted to take part. This resulted in a very positive experience: the girls were keen to talk about their sex education, but explained that boys would tease them if they volunteered. Adapting the way in which focus groups were carried out and working with the teachers involved enabled these girls' views to be included.

Similarly, after carrying out focus groups with students from the first cohort of the study, we felt concerned that we were not hearing from the 'quiet' students. We decided to try some interviews with pairs of 'quiet' students, but these were of mixed success. In general, students seemed intimidated by this, possibly because they did not choose to take part (they were usually asked by teachers and probably found it difficult to say no). Most research has to struggle with the challenge of reaching and engaging reticent participants, though research in school settings may see reticence amplified because of the power structures of the school. As researchers we have had to develop a sensitivity to the social context of the research and the school, and devise ways of working with teachers and identifying additional resources in order to get the 'best' contexts for as wide a range of views as possible.

Taking account of the context: issues relating to classroom culture and practices

Some of the ways in which aspects of the school context have influenced our use of methods have already been discussed – for example, the recruitment of volunteers for focus groups, and use of support teachers to help with questionnaire completion. Throughout the RIPPLE study it has been clear that the interaction between school practices and research methods has enormous significance in terms of the data obtained; the importance of working with teachers and ensuring they have a clear understanding of the aims of particular research activities cannot be overstated. An example is providing a clear explanation of the importance of providing all students with an opportunity to fill in the questionnaire. This involves explaining why non-completers and non-attenders may be particularly important for the study, because they may be at high risk in terms of adverse sexual health outcomes. Taking teachers through these explanations meant they were able to ensure that more people had the opportunity to take part. Where students might previously have been removed from classes if they were perceived as being disruptive or unable to answer the questions, teachers could take steps to ensure they were included. Similarly, involvement in the research motivated teachers to find time for students who were absent when we visited the school. Without teachers' engagement with the study these students' views would not be represented in the study data.

At times, aspects of school culture conflicted with attempts to include and engage students in the research and to access their views. For example, the use of discipline and authority sometimes obstructed the desired classroom conditions for the research. In their address to students, teachers would sometimes demand silence and diligence when completing questionnaires, and exert discipline over misdemeanours such as chewing gum or wearing a coat in the classroom. On occasions teachers would walk up and down aisles, creating unease for some students completing the questionnaires. In some instances, teachers elevated our status as researchers in the classroom by over-emphasizing our importance and urging students to behave courteously and with respect. This placed us in a difficult position. We were aware that we might be contradicting the teacher in our attempts to defuse the sometimes censorious atmosphere and create a more equal relationship between ourselves and the students, and convey to students that their participation was entirely voluntary, and we wanted honest and accurate data.

On other occasions, some students' expectations of the classroom experience led them to treat the researcher and the research with suspicion. Because of this, researchers found it difficult to gain cooperation and had to resort to 'teacher-like' discipline in order to address the class. It may well be that the classroom and even the school may not be the best context for collecting the views of some students.

How methods and context influence the data gathered

Gathering data on participants' responses to different methodologies is invaluable, and in the RIPPLE study has enabled us to develop more appropriate and sensitive methods. In addition, by collecting information about the ways in which these methods work in the school context we have been able to consider in turn how this context may influence the kind of data obtained. These reflections will feed into conclusions about the generalizability of the RIPPLE findings to other populations and contexts.

Analysis of students' questionnaire comments indicates that the act of completing the questionnaire may itself influence people's feelings about themselves and issues related to sex: for example, 'The questionnaire was good and made me know more about myself', or 'Thank you for this questionnaire. It has made me x-press my inner feelings.' In this sense, taking part in research may have an influence on the attitudes and behaviours being measured.

Likewise, fieldnotes from the sex education observed by researchers give insight into the extent to which researchers' presence may have influenced the process and outcomes of the study. During sessions, researchers were sometimes consulted about various parts of the lesson: for example, in several classes year 12 peer-educators checked factual information they were unsure about with the researcher. On occasions, the researcher would catch the eye of a particular student when an event occurred: for example, a year 9 student gauging the researcher's reaction when using sexually explicit language. The fieldnotes do not suggest that interactions between year 9 students were obviously censored by the presence of a researcher. Students spoke candidly with their peers and with the peer educators and in most instances seemed to pay little attention to the researcher. Anonymous questionnaires completed by year 12 peer educators after they had delivered the sessions asked, 'How did you feel about the researcher's presence throughout the project?' Only one person of the 151 people responding in the first cohort felt uncomfortable with researchers' presence; most said they felt comfortable or okay, while 18 said that they had been unaware of the researcher's presence.

Discussion

There are numerous reasons for integrating 'qualitative' methods and collecting 'qualitative' data as part of a 'quantitative' experimental research design. Three of the main justifications are: that such strategies can increase the likelihood of a trial reflecting the issues that are of greatest importance to the people involved; that they will help to ensure high participation and response rates; and that without them the research will have gained very little understanding of the processes involved in implementing an intervention, or of how social contexts are affected by, and themselves affect, research.

What follows summarizes some of the important issues that have arisen over the past two years, and includes some suggestions for things that could be done differently.

- *Evaluating research methods.* Collecting information from the students on research methods has been useful to develop these methods and our ways of deploying them so that they can best access young people's views. Although time-consuming, documenting issues that arise when using different methods provides important information about the influence of methods and context on the data obtained.
- *Using context-specific research methods.* The success of research methods in accessing people's views is dependent on these being appropriate to the context. A greater awareness of the school culture allows us to make predictions about the ways in which students can be recruited to take part, where research activities would best be held (e.g. more informal

settings, outside of the classroom), the kind of issues that need to be addressed when explaining research (e.g. confidentiality and the role of the researcher).

- *Working with teachers.* If teachers understand the aims of the research and particular methods they are able to ensure that the views of marginalized students can be reached (e.g. through following up absentees). Teachers are also in a position to advise on which methods and approaches are most likely to be the most effective (although they are not always right).
- *Establishing an open relationship with students.* This requires clear explanations of the overall aims of the research and of particular aspects of the process (e.g. why we ask particular questions). Such explanations allow students to make an informed choice to participate, and increase the likelihood of them being engaged and thus taking part in the process. However, providing explanations requires adequate time and resources.
- *Focusing on those whose views may be marginalized.* This requires sensitivity to those whose views may not be being heard, for whatever reason. Alternative ways in which these views might be accessed need to be considered.
- *Using a range of research tools.* These need to be relevant and inclusive, and capable of reflecting a variety of opinions and views from key stakeholders in the research project.

Conclusions

Although there is an increasing discussion about the desirability of integrating different research methods, there are few well worked examples of this in practice. Most RCTs in the health care field do not make use of methods such as observation and focus groups, nor do they prioritize the need to access participants' views fully. Applying RCT designs to social or behavioural interventions is by no means a new art (Oakley 1998b), nor is it as contentious as some would make out (Stephenson and Imrie 1998), but it does pose particular challenges. Combining methods within a trial design can be very labour-intensive, and expensive in terms of data handling: for example, coding free-text and transcribing tapes of interviews or focus groups. All the methods described in this chapter have been implemented by three researchers (two full-time, one part-time), working with 8,000 young people and around 130 staff in 27 schools. But it can equally be expensive to undertake trials without collecting such data, thereby making it impossible to answer key research questions.

A particular challenge is to move beyond the usual practice of combining methods, in which 'qualitative' data are analysed separately and sit alongside 'quantitative' measures of outcome. For example, in the RIPPLE study the observational data are being coded to create variables which describe the implementation and acceptability of the intervention. These variables and data will then be entered into the computer database and analysed integrally with the 'quantitative' data. Yet, however creative the procedures researchers can develop, there may remain a certain tension between the principles of a standardized intervention tested in an RCT and the notion of 'listening' to a whole community of research participants. An intervention that is standardized across different settings and time periods is, by definition, not one that is being constantly adapted to the needs of particular research participants. This tension between 'objectivity' and 'sensitivity' is one of the most interesting aspects of the RIPPLE study.

Acknowledgements

The RIPPLE study team comprises the authors of this chapter, Professor Ann Johnson, Dr Judith Stephenson, Stephanie Black and Angela Flux (State of Flux). Those formerly involved include Susan Charleston and Gayle Johnson.

We would like to thank the schools and the young people attending them for their support of the project and active participation in helping us to reflect on our research practice and build constructively on our experiences. Our thanks also go to all the people who helped us to conduct the questionnaire surveys described in this chapter. Without their preparedness to keep anti-social hours and represent the research team in classrooms the study would not have been possible. Finally, thank you to Susan Charleston who was involved in writing the first draft of this chapter. The RIPPLE project is funded by the Medical Research Council (MRC).

References

Basch, C. E. (1987) Focus group interview: an underutilized research technique for improving theory and practice in health education. *Health Education Quarterly*, 14(4), 411–48.
Burgess, R. G. (1983) *Experiencing Comprehensive Education: A Study of Comprehensive Education*. London: Methuen.
Department of Health (1992) *The Health of the Nation*. London: HMSO.
Davies, J. K. and Macdonald, G. (1998) *Quality, Evidence and Effectiveness in Health Promotion*. London: Routledge.
Fennell, R. (1993) A review of evaluations of peer education programs. *Journal of American College Health*, 41(6), 251–3.
Green, L. and Kreuter, W. (1991) *Health Promotion Planning: An Educational and Environmental Approach*. Mountain View, CA: Mayfield Publishing.
Hunter, D. (1993) Let's hear it for R&D. *Health Service Journal*, 15 April, 17.
Johnson, A. M., Wadsworth, J., Wellings, K. and Field, J. (1994) *Sexual Attitudes and Lifestyles, British Survey*. London: Blackwell Scientific Press.
Kitzinger, J. (1995) The methodology of focus groups: the importance of interaction between research participants. *Sociology of Health and Illness*, 16(1), 103–21.

Lawrence, J., Kanabus, A. and Regis, D. (2000) *A Survey of Sex Education Provision in Secondary Schools*. Horsham: AVERT.

Mathie, E. and Ford, N. (1994) *Evaluation of a College-based HIV and Sexual Health Peer Education Project in Somerset. Year One: A Summary*. Exeter: University of Exeter, Institute of Population Studies.

Moore, H. and Kindness, L. (1998) Establishing a research agenda for the health and wellbeing of children and young people in the context of health promotion. In A. Moore and Executive Working Group (eds) *Promoting the Health of Children and Young People: Setting a Research Agenda*. London: Health Education Authority.

Oakley, A. (1998a) Gender, methodology and people's ways of knowing: some problems with feminism and the paradigm debate in social science. *Sociology*, 32(4), 707–31.

Oakley, A. (1998b) Experimentation in social science: the case of health promotion. *Social Sciences in Health*, 4(2), 73–89.

Oakley, A. (2000) *Experiments in Knowing: Gender and Method in the Social Sciences*. Cambridge: Polity Press.

Oakley, A. and Fullerton, D. (1996) The lamppost of research: support or illumination? In A. Oakley and H. Roberts (eds) *Evaluating Social Interventions*. Ilford: Barnardo's.

Oakley, A., Fullerton, D., Holland J. *et al.* (1995) Sexual health interventions for young people: a methodological review. *British Medical Journal*, 310, 158–62.

Pearson, D. (1999) Sex education policies in schools: the first hurdle. *Health Education*, 99(3), 110–15.

Robson, C. (1993) *Real World Research*. Oxford: Blackwell.

Scott, S. (1992) Evaluation may change your life, but it won't solve all your problems. In P. Aggleton, P. Young, D. Moody, M. Kapila and M. Pye (eds) *Does It Work? Perspectives on the Evaluation of HIV/AIDS Health Promotion*. London: Health Education Authority.

Social Exclusion Unit (1999) *Teenage Pregnancy*. London: Cabinet Office Social Exclusion Unit.

Spradley, J. P. (1980) *Participant Observation*. New York: Rinehart and Winston.

Stenhouse, L. (1982) The conduct, analysis and reporting of case study in educational research and evaluation. In R. McCormick (ed.) *Calling Education to Account*. London: Heinemann.

Stephenson, J. M. and Imrie, J. (1998) Why do we need randomised controlled trials to assess behavioural interventions? *British Medical Journal*, 315, 611–13.

Stephenson, J. M., Oakley, A., Charleston, S. *et al.* (1998) Behavioural intervention trials for HIV/STD prevention in schools: are they feasible? *Sexually Transmitted Infections*, 74, 405–8.

Weston, R. (1998) Intertexuality: the current historical context of health promotion, cancer prevention and evaluation. In R. Weston and D. Scott (eds) *Evaluating Health Promotion*. Cheltenham: Stanley Thornes.

Williams, G. and Popay, J. (1997) Social science and public health: issues of method, knowledge and power. *Critical Public Health*, 7(1/2), 61–72.

▶ **Part 4**

▷ Advances in evidence-informed policy
and practice

▶ **11**

▷ # Using research: challenges in evidence-informed service planning

▷ ## Sandy Oliver, Greet Peersman, Ann Oakley and Amanda Nicholas

This chapter tells the story of how a group of health promotion specialists embarked on an evidence-based approach to health promotion and how they responded to the challenges. Their opportunity came through an invitation from the EPPI-Centre in 1996 to a series of workshops designed to support 'Promoting Health after Sifting the Evidence' (PHASE). The invitation was a direct result of Department of Health funding to encourage evidence-based health promotion and was an extension of the significant movement over the past ten years towards evidence-based medicine, which challenges the dominant role played by subjectivity in medical decision-making (Sackett *et al.* 1995; Maynard and Chalmers 1997). This new emphasis on the need for health care decisions to be informed by reliable evidence of effectiveness has spread to other areas, so that we now have calls for evidence-based policy (Ham *et al.* 1995), evidence-based purchasing (Fahey *et al.* 1995) and, indeed, evidence-based everything (Editorial Choice 1995).

Aside from the academic debate about appropriate methodologies for health promotion (see Chapters 1 and 2), commissioners and providers of health promotion services do in practice ask fundamental questions about the value of the work they support. Which interventions are effective and how do we know? What are the most efficient ways of finding the most reliable evidence? However, much health promotion work is supported without these questions being addressed. There are many reasons why this happens, but the difficulty of accessing relevant and appropriate research evidence and the lack of skills to judge quickly whether this is reliable and applicable to current, local needs are important factors.

The PHASE workshops were an innovative project designed to develop critical appraisal skills among health promotion specialists. The aims of the PHASE project were: (a) to raise awareness of the need to base health promotion interventions on reliable evidence about their effectiveness; (b) to disseminate sources of effectiveness data; and (c) to improve skills in critical appraisal among those working in the field of health promotion. In the event, the workshops unearthed a variety of other barriers that needed to be overcome to facilitate the use of research in the decision-making process.

Collaboration between researchers and service providers in developing PHASE

The PHASE workshops were based on the Critical Appraisal Skills Programme (CASP) developed by the Oxford Institute of Health Sciences, a practical and accessible programme for applying the principles and practice of evidence-based medicine (Milne *et al.* 1995). The CASP programme was designed originally for purchasers of health care and subsequently for the specific needs of other decision-makers in the National Health Service (NHS). A series of five PHASE workshops was developed by drawing on the extensive experience of CASP with multidisciplinary groups, and adapted specifically for health promotion with the help of prospective workshop participants and their peers.[1] Planning meetings with purchasers and providers were spread over five months. These meetings discussed: the potential relevance of critical appraisal to the work of purchasers and providers; the choice of topics and practical problems on which to centre the learning; and opportunities for prospective participants to take leading roles in the delivery of the workshops.

Effective Health Care Bulletins and the *Cochrane Database of Systematic Reviews* (the product of an international collaborative effort to review systematically evidence of effectiveness of health services, published as part of The Cochrane Library) were primary sources of research reports (see Chapters 3, 4 and 7) for critical appraisal in the workshops. These reports were chosen to reflect an interest in peer-led programmes and community development identified during the planning meetings. However, the finding of sufficient research papers which would satisfy workshop participants was hampered by the dearth of sound evaluations of effectiveness in health promotion. Another constraint was the importance paid by many health promotion providers to criteria such as the degree of community participation in judging the quality of interventions (Speller *et al.* 1997). Again, the literature here is not well developed. The series of workshops addressed the following research areas: an investigation of the diffusion of an anti-smoking programme through a school system; a trial of peer sex education in schools; a randomized controlled trial of AIDS education interventions for homosexually active men; a systematic review of smoking cessation programmes for pregnant women; and a proposal for evaluating an accident prevention intervention aimed at mothers with young children. An additional workshop focused on the appraisal of a proposal for evaluating a sexual health promotion outreach programme prepared by a workshop participant.

Health promotion specialists provide services in the voluntary, as well as the statutory, sector. NHS health authorities purchase their services on behalf of their local populations and may influence whether and how services are delivered through purchasing contracts with service providers. Hence, the PHASE workshops were aimed at both purchasers and providers. Because the EPPI-Centre was partly funded to carry out work in the area of evaluating sexual health promotion, there was an emphasis on this speciality in inviting participants. Individuals with responsibility for purchasing or providing sexual health promotion services within the North Thames Regional Health Authority were invited, as were others throughout England and Wales. The letters with flyers advertising the series of six workshops emphasized the value of attending more than one workshop in the series.

Considerable effort was expended in designing the workshop materials: adopting non-medical language; addressing different stages in working towards evidence-based services; determining what information different research designs are likely to yield; investigating both processes and outcomes. Materials were sent to participants one week in advance of the workshop and contained an introduction to the concept of evidence-based health promotion and the paper for appraisal during the workshop.

The workshops were set up as interactive sessions designed to learn about others' ideas and expertise. Each workshop lasted for four to five hours and was divided into four parts: (a) a plenary session which introduced key concepts for learning from reports of feasibility, acceptability and effectiveness in health promotion; (b) critical appraisal of a research paper in small groups; (c) participants sharing the discussions and conclusions from their small group work in a plenary session and considering the opportunities to apply critical appraisal skills in their work; and (d) a short evaluation session, with a questionnaire and group discussion. Each workshop was delivered by a team of researchers and health promotion purchasers and providers.

The workshops were held in London: nearly half the participants worked in London, and had an interest in sexual health promotion services. Over half the places were taken by providers of health promotion services, with most of the remainder being equally divided between purchasers of services and those with responsibilities for both purchasing and providing; there were very few people from the voluntary sector or academic institutions.

Facing a challenge

Despite efforts to adapt the workshops to suit health promotion needs, with considerable help from health promotion specialists in both the development and delivery of the workshops, participants still faced serious hurdles before they were ready to consider and adopt evidence-based approaches.

At the start of the workshops, most participants indicated that they had, in the course of their work, asked questions about the availability, acceptability and effectiveness of particular health promotion approaches and programmes, but only half of them had found an answer; those who had, had referred mainly to the opinions of their immediate colleagues, internal reports or personal experience. This reliance on professional opinions rather than published sources of information about effectiveness of health promotion has been reported in other studies of professional decision-making (Shadish and Epstein 1987; Bonell 1996). Many health promotion providers either did not have access to, or chose not to use, sources of information which specialize in reliable evidence of effectiveness, such as the Effective Health Care Bulletins produced by the Centre for Reviews and Dissemination in York and the *Cochrane Database of Systematic Reviews* produced by the Cochrane Collaboration.

Some workshop participants were sceptical of Effective Health Care Bulletins as an appropriate and useful source of information for health promotion, with their emphasis on the use of randomized controlled trials (RCTs). Over the past few years, the 'anti-positivism' of some health promotion practitioners and researchers has had to deal with weighty evidence that design matters in this field, but the debate about what constitutes appropriate evaluation in health promotion lingers (see Chapter 2). Even when participants would like to address the issue of effectiveness of health promotion, they could be 'bowed down trying to demonstrate the effectiveness of what they're doing', and claimed that 'research is actually the last thing used to make a decision in the current political climate.'

One participant explained the difficulties of trying to base work on research evidence:

> I often find myself in the position of asking questions like these . . . and *either* not really having the time/resources/skills to look for answers *or* assuming that there are no answers and trying to work out how we can find them from scratch, e.g. focus groups on new resources, pre–post course questionnaires for training programmes. Sometimes the latter response is well founded. Working in a relatively well funded, large, inner-London Health Promotion Service, we are often in the forefront of work. When I look elsewhere for relevant information for training, condom distribution etc. I've found little that is inspiring . . . But clearly there are times when I'm not aware of what is available, relevant or of how to access this material. It is the latter point that really worries me.

A recurrent theme of discussion throughout the series was the desired balance between building the research skills of practitioners and commissioners and their acquisition of research-based information. Ironically for a profession espousing the empowerment of others (see Chapter 1), many of them rejected the opportunity to empower themselves with new skills. They would have preferred to be told what was effective rather than apply their own judgement to a report: 'People want critical appraisal done for them, not to do it themselves – some people struggle with the conceptual understanding and the statistics.' Nevertheless, some rose to the challenge: 'I thought I would learn about good practice, not the process of how to find good practice – nevertheless this is beneficial and I think I learned this. I would have liked to come to all five.'

Needs for research training

Some participants were very clear about their needs for support and information when working towards effective health promotion. Some wanted information on what studies or papers are available and on current work in their particular topic area, and advice on what they were proposing to do – was it effective or how could they make it more effective? Some wanted discussion: 'I think most health promotion staff have skills to appraise an article. What is needed is an overview of evidence in specific areas, e.g. smoking. [We need] a consensus on what can be taken from [the evidence] and [the recommended] programmes.' Others wanted support in developing and evaluating their own work:

> [We need] discussion and 'refereeing' of project evaluation planning before rather than after the event [and] techniques for presenting the case for valid and effective evaluation in the context of multi-agency projects where consensus issues must be addressed.

> I need a follow-up workshop to help me design an intervention. I need help in developing my own skills – either a workshop or other support.

Some participants wanted to share their newly acquired skills with their colleagues. Others planned to use the critical appraisal guidelines for their own report writing. This may lead to more clarity about the research questions and conclusions of internal reports, which is particularly encouraging because health promotion has a wealth of 'grey literature' evaluation reports that are often not widely or systematically disseminated, and hence are difficult to obtain for inclusion in for example, systematic reviews (see Chapters 7 and 8).

Barriers to a concerted solution

Just like the individual behaviour change interventions for healthy lifestyles, any individual changes in attitudes towards using research are unlikely to reap real benefits without facilitative changes in the working environment. The opportunity for workshop learning to improve effectiveness in practice was impeded by the organizational structure of the NHS internal market, a structure ultimately aimed at improving services. The need for services to secure funding from commissioners proved to be a barrier to open discussion in workshops:

> There was a provider commissioner divide [in the workshops] – some health promotion managers were defensive. [Despite this] the debate and evaluation was useful and the most interesting part of the day.

> Agencies are set up in competition so it's difficult.

The fact that some providers were reluctant to share their ideas with competing provider units is yet another barrier to sharing each other's resources and expertise, which needs to be addressed by purchasers and providers together. However, learning together is possible and can be very productive, as was experienced within the relaxed atmosphere of a subsequent specially commissioned PHASE workshop held outside London, where participants knew each other and were used to meeting regularly. They particularly valued:

> an opportunity to explore and discuss evaluation with colleagues in a focused setting.

> discussions, sharing with colleagues, [the] process of being together.

> the time it permitted us as a group to discuss evaluation issues.

> the opportunity to share concerns, issues and fears with colleagues.

In addition to potential barriers to open discussion, the pressures imposed by contracting cycles within the NHS were brought forward as a problem with using research in the decision-making process. Participants discussed these barriers and the need for providing an environment that is conducive to integrating research and practice:

> [There is a] time pressure on reading, reflecting, and processing evaluation reports.

> [We need] an environment where evaluation is supported. At the moment all good intentions are hopelessly unrealistic.

> [We need] the time to do it within a contract.

> People need to know it's OK to spend a day in the library . . . searching properly.

It was clear that a concerted effort was called for involving all those working towards effective health promotion:

We need to clarify a legitimate role for commissioners in stimulating and funding research. We need to clarify a legitimate role for providers. And to analyse the relationship between research and practice and the potential for incorporating research into practice.

However, the complementary aim of incorporating research into practice, in other words developing services in a research framework when the evidence is lacking, still seemed a little far-fetched:

> I have a very positive attitude to evaluating health promotion and debating RCTs etc., but I feel there has been a push that RCTs are essential and a lack of acknowledgement that health promotion specialists cannot do this ... I am all for critical appraisal but the reality is that RCTs aren't out there and we are not resourced to undertake them. This has to be acknowledged and discussed further.

An important finding was that even enthusiasts of evidence-based health promotion are demotivated by the lack of support and resources for evaluation and the restrictions imposed by the contracting/commissioning cycle. In an environment that advocates evaluation and using research in the decision-making process, contracts need to allow time for literature searches to inform new projects and for the planning of interventions to include appropriate evaluation.

Collaborative moves towards evidence-based health promotion

PHASE workshops acted as a catalyst for raising awareness of evidence-based health promotion among practitioners, provided a forum for people with different skills and vested interests to consider how to circumnavigate constraints in moving towards evidence-based practice and indicated opportunities for harnessing research to the needs of services and clients. Health promotion specialists need quick access to the research literature, and want to find evaluations that accommodate the principles that they espouse in their work: a holistic attitude to health and interventions benefiting from the insights of all concerned.

The EPPI-Centre website can be the catalyst for taking some of these issues forward. In order to answer pragmatic questions of effectiveness and appropriateness relevant to the current enthusiasm for interventions built on community development or healthy alliances, there is a need to search systematically for outcome evaluations of 'healthy alliances' and review such studies both for the degree and quality of community participation and for evidence of effectiveness. This has been taken on board by the EPPI-Centre in preparing reviews of 'healthy alliances' that are a part of workplace health promotion interventions (Peersman *et al.* 1998) and peer-delivered interventions for young people (see Chapter 8). Many interventions and evaluations have conventionally focused more on targeting specific health problems than on influencing the broad range of health measures, encompassing psycho-social outcomes, favoured by most health promotion specialists. Chapter 12 describes how the scope of a systematic review has been broadened with the help of health promotion practitioners and service users, with consequences for planning services, evaluating existing interventions and developing new ones.

Each group working in health promotion has developed skills and priorities to make the most progress within its own arena. But making progress independently from others in the field is problematic, as the urgency of health needs may not coincide with settings most amenable to investigation, and realizing the ultimate aim of improving health may be frustrated by both irrelevant research and services with unknown impact (Nutbeam 1996). While practitioners and their local populations may share with researchers the ultimate aim of promoting health appropriately and cost-effectively, conflicts of interest may arise because practitioners, researchers and the populations they serve direct their efforts at different stages in the development process, and work within different constraints. The contribution of the local populations is often limited by the time and effort they can afford to give voluntarily. The contribution of practitioners may be driven by political imperatives at a national or local level, and researchers attract funding for their contribution on the strength of their research methodology.

Developing and delivering health promotion services that are both appropriate and effective requires knowledge about the health needs of local populations, the skills and resources required and available for the services, and their impact. Health promotion practitioners are sufficiently close to working with their local populations to assess health needs and elicit preferences and criteria for success. Piloting interventions, examining service delivery, acceptability and impact, may be carried out in collaboration with researchers. Involving the community is not an alternative to evaluating effectiveness but a necessary part of evaluating effectiveness well. Healthy alliances and evidence-based health are not mutually exclusive, but complementary approaches which extend the principle of involving stakeholders to decision-making at all stages of the research process: from needs assessment and developing services to evaluating interventions and systematically reviewing the research literature. Community development will be particularly well informed if it begins with communities appraising the literature themselves, as some lay organizations are already doing (Milne and Oliver 1996). They may access literature with the help of the EPPI-Centre website and appraise what they find with PHASE critical appraisal tools.

Conclusions

The key messages from this chapter are:

- Health promotion specialists can develop skills to use research literature, but they need a conducive working environment.
- Health promotion funders can encourage evidence-based services by allowing time and resources for seeking and appraising literature to inform service planning and by funding interventions with integrated evaluations.
- In using research, effectiveness studies need to be integrated with the principles of community development and 'health for all'.

Note

1 CASP, at the Oxford Institute of Health Sciences, has since developed workshops specifically for health promotion and these are still available.

References

Bonell, C. (1996) *Outcomes in HIV Prevention: Report of a Research Project.* London: The HIV Project.

Editorial Choice (1995) Celebrating evidence-based everything. *British Medical Journal*, 310.

Fahey, T., Griffiths, S. and Peters, T. J. (1995) Evidence-based purchasing: understanding results of clinical trials and systematic reviews. *British Medical Journal*, 311, 1056–9.

Ham, C., Hunter, D. J. and Robinson, R. (1995) Evidence-based policy making. *British Medical Journal*, 310, 71–2.

Lumley, J. (1993) Stategies for reducing smoking in pregnancy. In J. Neilson *et al.* (eds) *Pregnancy and Childbirth Module of the Cochrane Database of Systematic Reviews* (updated 27 September). Available in the Cochrane Pregnancy and Childbirth Database, 1995, Issue 1.

Maynard, A. and Chalmers, I. (eds) (1997) *Non-random Reflections on Health Services Research.* London: BMJ Publishing Group.

Milne, R., Donald, A. and Chambers, L. (1995) Piloting short workshops on the critical appraisal of reviews. *Health Trends*, 27(4), 120–3.

Milne, R. and Oliver, S. (1996) Evidence-based consumer health information: developing trends in critical appraisal skills. *International Journal for Quality in Health Care*, 8(5), 439–45.

Peersman, G., Harden, A. and Oliver, S. (1998) *Effectiveness of Health Promotion Interventions in the Workplace: A Review.* London: Health Education Authority.

Nutbeam, D. (1996) Achieving 'best practice' in health promotion: improving the fit between research and practice. *Health Education Research*, 11, 317–26.

Sackett, D. L., Rosenburg, W. M. C., Gray, J. A. M., Haynes, R. B. and Richardson, W. S. (1995) Evidence-based medicine: what it is and what it isn't. *British Medical Journal*, 312, 71–2.

Shadish, W. R. and Epstein, R. (1987) Patterns of program evaluation practice among members of the Evaluation Research Society and Evaluation network. *Evaluation Review*, 11, 555–90.

Speller, V., Learmonth, A. and Harrison, D. (1997) The search for evidence of effective health promotion. *British Medical Journal*, 315, 361–3.

▷ Making research more useful: integrating different perspectives and different methods

▷ **Sandy Oliver**

Fresh perspectives can radically alter understanding

For centuries it has been widely held that Oliver Cromwell's appalling atrocities in 1649 included a massacre of the unarmed citizens of Drogheda: men and women, old people and children. This story has now been refuted by the owner of a local software recycling company who has delved into contemporary documents (Reilly 1999). As an amateur historian he has a love for his subject and fresh eyes, 'he is scrupulous in his examination of evidence, he has necessary scepticism, he is assiduous in research and quotes primary material extensively' (Edwards 1999).

Another example of received wisdom being turned upside down is the character of Chaucer's Knight, long believed to be the pinnacle of honour and good breeding, who comes first in the sequence of pilgrims because he is the standard by which the others should be judged (Sillars 1983). It was Terry Jones, graduate in English and comedian, who proposed that the Knight's portrait is a piece of sustained irony which is intended to suggest an evil and corrupt nature (Jones 1985). Jones turned away from books of literary criticism and was inspired by history books and a tourist guide book of Doune Castle picked up while filming *Monty Python and the Holy Grail*. He drew on another discipline to advance ideas of literary criticism.

The historical interpretation of Cromwell in Ireland and the literary interpretation of Chaucer's Knight are controversial; neither longstanding subject experts nor newcomers can be assumed to have a monopoly of the truth. Newcomers, whether drawing on a different discipline or coming from a different occupation, are particularly valuable because they are constrained neither by conventional disciplinary boundaries nor by the assumptions of a formal training and, without a professional reputation to defend, they can afford to propose apparently outlandish ideas. The results are very thought provoking.

History and literature are particularly open to review because many people have first hand experience of both. Similarly with health. We all experience health: good health, bad health or both; and we all experience health care, whether caring for ourselves or caring for others in a professional or personal capacity. Thus, in theory, health and health care are particularly open to advances because they are open to contributions from many perspectives. However, most people's potential for influence is curbed because although in the private domain they learn, teach and care for themselves and others on a daily basis, in the public domain health, social and educational services have been reserved predominantly for the influence of a limited circle of professionals. For instance, it is widely recognized that health care has become professionalized, with the efforts of the most numerous health care providers, mothers, being almost invisible and largely ignored in decisions about health care and health care research. Because health is medicalized and professionalized, resistance to radical new ideas is enormous.

Perspectives in health promotion

Health promotion is currently experiencing controversies between the different approaches of public health, 'Health for All' and self-help. People in these three spheres are inspired by deeply held ethical principles. Medically dominated public health was quick to adopt the principles of effectiveness in health care; 'Health for All' particularly values community participation; and the right to information and choice is claimed by a wide range of consumer organizations. Although these principles are not mutually exclusive, how they have been pursued by their different protagonists has created divisions.

Evidence-based health has grown from the writing of Archie Cochrane, who marched in the 1930s under the banner of 'All effective care should be free' and subsequently advocated increasing rigour in the measurement of effectiveness (Cochrane 1972). Health promotion today emphasizes ways of involving communities in identifying both health problems and strategies for addressing those problems (Minkler 1989). With a trend in developed countries away from institutional help towards self-help and from representative democracy towards participative democracy, communities and self-help groups are taking the initiative to improve health through campaigning for services and developing self-reliant alternatives (Naisbitt 1982). These include housing associations and owner-builders for their homes, neighbourhood watch for tackling crime and support groups for a myriad of disadvantages and misadventures. Greater information and self-determination for patients and the general public are their guiding principles.

These movements have developed strong identities through their separate histories and often challenged each other's assumptions, rather than combined their different experiences and principles to forge new ideas. Medicine and public health have exposed and redressed a complacency about intervention research whereby claims of effectiveness by practitioners have been made and acted upon in the absence of rigorous evidence. Health promotion, on the other hand, has employed 'action research' to develop complex community interventions which present particular challenges to evaluation of their effects. It has also stressed the importance of involving ordinary people in identifying their health needs, although often in a consultative capacity which can be seen as paternalistic, despite a rhetoric of 'empowerment' (Peersman 1999). 'Empowered' consumers and their advocates have emphasized not 'need', as in health promotion, but people's 'rights'; and 'care' and 'coping' as well as 'cure'. Calls for care and coping to be considered as well as cure particularly challenge health treatment services because they require health to be considered in terms of everyday living rather than in terms of signs and symptoms of illness and use of services. This is a challenge not only to the services, but also to the research which should be informing the development of those services.

Empowerment in research

One route to resolving these controversies is to fuse the efforts of practioners, researchers and health service consumers, including the public, to change how research is conducted, and consequently the knowledge created, as well as how it is used (see Chapter 9).

In practice, consumers can be found influencing research both at the invitation of professionals and, more radically, as part of their peer support and campaigning activities. For instance, one joint venture brought together the Social Services Inspectorate of the Department of Health and Arthritis Care. Their aim was to improve community services for isolated disabled people (Minkes et al. 1995). Arthritis Care provided members of the project team and 40 individuals were selected for interview through the Arthritis Care local networks. The Social Services Inspectorate provided other members of the project team, analysis of the interview schedules and an independent consultant to write the report. Other alliances have been between different consumer groups, such as a study of poverty and undernourishment in pregnancy. This was undertaken by the Maternity Alliance, 'an educational and research trust working to make life better for pregnant women, new parents and their babies' and NCH Action for Sick Children, 'one of Britain's largest childcare charities, caring for many thousands of children in need and their families through 235 projects nation-wide' (Bloom 1993).

Consumers participate in, and sometimes lead, many types of studies: assessing health needs; eliciting views about services; piloting and evaluating new policies and services; and assessing the effectiveness of care through controlled trials or systematic reviews. These activities can be found across the range of public and private sectors, in research focusing on agriculture (Mills and Karanja 1997), child care and protection (Save the Children 1995), disability (Brienza et al. 1995), the environment (Phillimore and Moffatt 1994; Bouma 1998; Hannah et al. 1998), food safety (Finn and Louviere 1992), homelessness (Cohen et al. 1999), learning difficulties (Minkes et al. 1995), marketing (Bloom 1993) and occupational safety and health (Fise 1992).

Consumer groups may assess needs through their own networks, responding to the concerns of members or enquirers, or they may conduct formal needs assessments on behalf of statutory authorities (UK Coalition of People Living with HIV and AIDS 1996), in partnership with researchers (Rice et al. 1994), statutory agencies (Social Services Inspectorate and Arthritis Care 1996) or other voluntary sector agencies (Maternity Alliance and NCH Action for Sick Children 1995).

In health promotion services, where people are often invited to contribute to formal assessments of their own health needs, the active involvement of consumers in assessing services is relatively rare. A notable exception combined the participatory principles of health promotion and the concept of effectiveness research in a multisite randomized controlled trial of a health education programme for coke oven workers in the American steel industry, which aimed to reduce the risk of occupational lung cancer (Parkinson et al. 1989). This involved a unique collaboration between academic researchers and the industry's trade union. The collaboration began eight years before the development of the intervention programme and affected the programme content and presentations, a publicity campaign, the design and content of questionnaires and telephone interview schedules, and the hiring and training of laid-off coke oven workers who served as telephone interviewers. All levels of the union were involved in the programme.

There are examples of consumer involvement in research across broad areas of health care – physical health, mental health, sexual health and social well-being – often with a particular emphasis on information and support needs. In particular, a few years ago, the Royal National Institute for the Blind (RNIB) asked parents of children who were blind and partially sighted how they thought the services and care they received could be improved. One of the things parents felt most strongly about was the lack of support and information at the time they were told about their child's sight problems. This provoked a subsequent investigation by RNIB workers of parents' experiences (Fise 1992).

Consumers have been involved in investigating prevention, treatment and support services, in the community, in primary care and in general or specialist hospital services. The charity Changing Faces is unusual in targeting its own services for investigation because it intends that all its work be underpinned, monitored and informed by objective research (Changing Faces 1995–6). In partnership with the Faculty of Community Studies, University of the West of England, Changing Faces evaluated the impact of its own programme of social interaction skills workshops to help adults to tackle the problems associated with facial disfigurement (Robinson *et al.* 1996). This is an example of consumer interests extending beyond the conventional scope of the NHS to include holistic approaches to health without artificial divisions of body systems or diseases, and multi-agency alliances.

I found most of the examples described above not by delving into professional research literature but by contacting consumer organizations and listening to their members talk about their campaigns, services and research. From such conversations I am repeatedly impressed by the valuable insights that consumers can bring to research and their holistic approaches to using research for problem-solving. I adopted a similarly broad approach, which spanned physical and mental well-being, and emphasized information and support, when I became involved in a systematic review of smoking cessation programmes for pregnant women. The review benefited enormously from the involvement of people from very different cultures: professional practitioners, lay carers, service users and the research community.

Criticism and collaboration

The rest of this chapter tells a story of this review. It is about crossing between cultures, the criticisms encountered, the opportunities for constructive collaboration and how this may change the nature of research and decisions about effectiveness. It highlights advances in research-based practice and practice-relevant research resulting from researchers, practitioners and service users working together; and illustrates how their different ideologies can advance research about effectiveness in which qualitative and experimental approaches to generating new knowledge are fully integrated and thereby more widely acceptable.

The issue at stake in this story is women smoking in pregnancy and how it should be addressed. Smoking in pregnancy has received attention from both evidence-based health and qualitative social research, with maternity research being more organized in the former and UK health promotion practitioners favouring the latter. On the one hand, smoking in pregnancy is a threat to women's and babies' physical health (it increases still birth and decreases birth weight) and is therefore a target for 'cure'. On the other hand, smoking, for disadvantaged women, particularly mothers, is also a way of coping with the stresses of poverty and isolation (Graham 1993), and is therefore a target for 'care'. The most common setting for addressing smoking in pregnancy is not in women's homes, where they cope with these pressures (or not), but in maternity and other health services. Here other controversies have raged between health professionals and consumer organizations about the medicalization of childbirth and rights to information and choice.

The meeting of research paradigms

When a stream of work at the EPPI-Centre was funded by the Department of Health in 1995 there was an explicit aim of bridging the gap between the rigorous research evidence of trials and systematic reviews, and what health promotion providers practice. This gap was readily apparent when we introduced systematic reviews of the effects of smoking cessation programmes in pregnancy (published in a pilot electronic journal, *The Cochrane Pregnancy and Childbirth Database*: Lumley 1995) to a workshop designed to encourage evidence-based health promotion (see Chapter 11). The reviews attracted strong criticism. The workshop participants were unimpressed by the reduction in smoking and increases in birth weights following interventions (Lumley 1995) when no account had been taken of family relationships. How could we know, they asked, whether on balance these programmes were beneficial if the evaluation ignored possible increases in stress in the mothers and their ability to cope calmly with their families? Might smoking cessation programmes also lead to children suffering or families breaking up as mothers' coping mechanisms were taken away? How could one justify implementing a programme with so little information? In addition, health promotion practitioners expressed concern about the practicalities of developing and delivering programmes. Were the programmes based on a theoretical understanding of behaviour? What did health professionals actually do, and did they do it well? Health promotion practitioners saw no value in combining the results of trials in a meta-analysis without taking these issues into account.

In an attempt to salvage the workshop in the face of a strong antipathy to these randomized controlled trials we invited participants to compose a letter to the author of the review suggesting how the systematic reviews could be improved. This they did. A letter was sent to the author from 14 workshop participants requesting that an update of the review include a clearer description of behavioural and other strategies for helping pregnant women to stop smoking, and that attention be drawn to the

> need for trials to address broader outcome measures such as the impact on other family members, the benefits to women's health, whether non-smoking is sustained, the impact of failing to stop smoking, stress levels, the emotional impact of having a low birth weight baby after

taking part in a strategy to stop smoking, and self-esteem, rather than having a merely medical focus on the baby.

(Letter to Lumley 1995)

These suggestions were sent in a 'supportive spirit of collaboration' and accepted as such by Judith Lumley, the author of the review.

Judith Lumley had also published qualitative social research about women smoking (Lumley 1991), so it was not surprising that she responded positively and promised to take their concerns into account when updating the work. In due course she invited me to join her in updating the review.

Women's contributions to systematic reviewing

Updating the review was also an opportunity to hear from other people with views on smoking, the women themselves. We sought women through what is formally called a rapid appraisal exercise, which in practice meant getting on the phone to mothers of small children who met regularly other mothers of small children, or approaching women in the school playground, and asking friends, family and neighbours. I asked about smoking, about quitting smoking and about not quitting smoking. We heard stories of easy success, painful failure, determination and indifference. While support and encouragement might motivate some women, others felt that their midwives' expressed concern about smoking during pregnancy marred their relationship, and midwives who offered unconditional emotional support to women who smoked were particularly appreciated. This is complicated further by some women's personal experience of health problems, or even tragedy, being more closely associated with quitting than smoking; for instance, when a woman lost her first baby despite quitting, but gave birth to a healthy second child after smoking throughout the pregnancy. Such wide variation in experience and attitudes is often mistakenly used as an argument for the futility of 'controlled trials' of social interventions. Ardent experimentalists, on the other hand, marvel at how randomizing individuals from a richly varied population into two or more groups is the most reliable method of matching groups (not individuals) and thereby accounting for human variety within experimentation. Less often, unfortunately, do they account for variety in the choice of outcomes adopted to assess the effects of intervening in people's lives. This is not an inherent problem of randomized controlled trials, and some triallists are now inviting consumers to join them in planning research (Hanley *et al.* 2001).

Methodological developments

Accepting these challenges meant amending the review methods to include more detail about the interventions and their delivery and to acknowledge a broad range of potential effects on babies and their mothers. We sought additional randomized controlled trials through the Cochrane Pregnancy and Childbirth Review Groups, and the Cochrane Tobacco Group, as was common practice. To ensure that the review was well informed about the nature and extent of the problem we drew on other studies, such as routinely collected state and national data, epidemiological surveys, surveys of professional practice, formative intervention studies, in-depth interviews and critical reviews. These descriptive and qualitative studies, together with discussions with health promotion practitioners and maternity service users, guided the review of evaluation reports. Bearing in mind the practitioners' need to know about how to replicate interventions, we systematically reviewed reports for information about who developed the interventions and how, whether the interventions had a theoretical basis, or took into account women's concerns, and how well their delivery was monitored. To evaluate the effects we collected data for a broad range of outcomes. We combined the results of the trials in a meta-analysis to estimate an average impact on smoking behaviour and health, and the review was published in the Cochrane Library (Lumley *et al.* 1998).

What more was learnt

General conclusions about the effects of smoking cessation programmes in pregnancy were clear. On average, smoking cessation programmes in pregnancy appeared to reduce smoking, low birth weight and preterm birth, but no effect was detected for very low birth weight or perinatal mortality. Smoking cessation was greatest with interventions that were particularly intense and had an explicit theoretical basis, and where the evaluation included a detailed description of the intervention sufficient for replication, a process evaluation and biochemically validated smoking cessation.

Reviewing process indicators explained some of the heterogeneity in outcomes: some interventions had been poorly delivered; if interventions were developed with one population they were not necessarily appropriate for another. Encouragingly, more intensive interventions showed a greater impact on smoking, as did those interventions based on theoretical understanding of behaviour.

However, reviewing studies from the perspective of service users revealed that outcomes which are important to women had been missed not only by systematic reviewers, but also by the original trialists. No trials reported any assessment of the impact of the intervention on the method of delivery, breast feeding, maternal psychological well-being or the well-being of other family members. It also showed that no studies reported a needs assessment which involved service users. Women's concerns about smoking as a coping mechanism, their anxiety about babies' size at delivery or the impact of their personal experience on their perception of risk associated with smoking were more often addressed in discussions following trial reports than in the design of interventions or their evaluation. Once these concerns are understood, there are opportunities to develop skills in coping strategies for everyday life, and additional support for women to help them cope in labour could be integrated into care programmes for women quitting smoking. A few studies had involved consumers in piloting the intervention, and some of these adapted materials in the light of this, but no studies explored the potential added value of involving service users in developing interventions.

This review shows how observational and qualitative research, and small-scale consultations, can influence the criteria by which the effectiveness of interventions are judged and, when reviewed systematically, reveal to what extent these criteria are adopted in policies and practice. Thus, discussing interventions and their evaluation with intervention specialists and health service users is important for informing a systematic review. Reviewing process indicators revealed information about the content, delivery and acceptability of interventions which is important for community uptake of the recommendations. These approaches to developing recommendations that are most relevant to current practice and research cross professional and disciplinary boundaries. They draw on the experiences of people using or working in health services as partners in research. Adapting review methods in the light of such consultations expands reviews of effects of care to address challenges to implementation and generate a broader research agenda.

This is not the only way to integrate ideas from different theoretical standpoints. A systematic review of effectiveness of workplace health promotion incorporated the views of practitioners and service users in other ways. The research team focused on those studies which had adhered to the principles of community involvement by basing interventions on what people felt was needed for their own health, or involving them in designing or evaluating interventions. Chapter 9 describes a similar approach taken to review peer-delivered health promotion interventions for young people which also drew on process evaluations to inform effectiveness in practice.

By engaging in dialogue, practitioners, researchers and service users have focused research on issues that matter more to the people most intimately affected by them – those receiving, missing or actively avoiding health promotion interventions. In doing so they have developed methods for considering care, cure and coping together.

So advocates for disadvantaged people and champions of qualitative research have inspired advances in systematic reviewing, a methodology predominantly led by doctors. We can see how the story has come full circle by reading the words of Archie Cochrane:

> I have devoted most of the . . . analysis of effectiveness and efficiency [to] cure, because so much more is known about it. There has been so little work done [about] 'care' . . . One is likely to breed bias when

dealing with medical treatment and medical care in the NHS ... In particular I believe that cure is rare while the need for care is widespread, and the pursuit of cure at all costs may restrict the supply of care.

Archie Cochrane knew more about the effectiveness of cure than care because he could draw on a raft of randomized controlled trials in medicine. His challenge to organize 'a critical summary, by speciality or sub-speciality, adapted periodically, of all relevant randomized controlled trials' (Cochrane 1979) was the catalyst for the new science of systematic reviewing. The greatest early advances were made in medicine. Systematic reviews of so-called 'complex' interventions, including health promotion, came later. Not that medicines are simple: their pharmacodynamics require careful and extensive research. But when the time comes to assess their effectiveness the intricacies of a pharmaceutical product and its potential to interact with ailing bodies are hidden within a sugar-coated pill, and single-minded attention is paid to the simple design of a randomized controlled trial.

It is not so with health promotion and other social interventions: even 'simple' interventions such as invitations for screening or leaflets advising healthy lifestyles are open to scrutiny throughout a trial. Is the layout of the leaflet appealing, is the language sensitive and how is it offered to potential readers? Do the readers embrace or ignore what is offered? If trials of leaflets with the same aims are considered in a single review, how reasonable is it to pool their results if the answers to these questions differ? The story of the smoking cessation review recounted above illustrates how questions about the design and the implementation of interventions can be taken into account when considering their effects. This approach can be extended to trials and systematic reviews in medicine. Who prescribes the medicine, what discussion precedes or follows and what does the packet insert say? Do patients embrace or ignore what is offered? If drug trials are considered in a single review, how reasonable is it to pool their results if the answers to these questions differ?

Health promotion has been forced to consider such complexities, to integrate theory, organization, performance and effectiveness. Now the way is open to apply these methods more widely. For this next step systematic reviewing, developed in medicine to assess achievements in cure, could learn some lessons developed in health promotion and give greater prominence to the social aspects of medicine in order to learn more about caring and coping.

Conclusions

This chapter demonstrates the importance of understanding the full picture when undertaking research: understanding who needs to know what and what sort of research can provide some answers. This includes the need to provide evidence of the effects of interventions, in terms acceptable to those on their receiving end as well as those delivering them, and information to guide the development and implementation of interventions. The story of the smoking cessation review also illustrates how this may be achieved with contributions from everyone involved. While researchers can design primary research and systematic reviews, including methods of data collection and analysis, the content of this work is better determined by those most intimately involved: practitioners, their clients and the wider public.

The key messages from this chapter are:

- The improvement of health and social welfare requires learning from practitioner and research experience, as well as health service consumers' experience.
- Looking at problems from different perspectives helps to identify what is required from research.
- Health service consumers can be empowered to influence research, including randomized controlled trials and systematic reviews.
- Actively involving practitioners and consumers in research can lead to advances in research methodology.

References

Bloom, P. N. (1993) Consumer research priorities for the MSI research competition on using marketing to serve society. *Advances in Consumer Research*, 20, 436.

Bouma, J. (1998) Realizing basic research in applied environmental research projects. *Journal of Environmental Quality*, 27(4), 742–9.

Brienza, D., Angelo, J. and Henry, K. (1995) Consumer participation in identifying research and development priorities for power wheelchair input devices and controllers. *Assistive-Technology*, 7(1), 55–62.

Changing Faces Annual Report, 1995–1996. London: Changing Faces.

Cochrane, A. L. (1972) *Effectiveness and Efficiency: Random Reflections on Health Services*. London: Nuffield Provincial Hospitals Trust.

Cochrane, A. L. (1979) 1931–1971: a critical review with particular reference to the medical profession. In *Medicines for the Year 2000*. London: Office of Health Economics.

Cohen, C. I., D'Onofrio, A., Larkin, L., Berkholder, P. and Fishman, H. (1999) A comparison of consumer and provider preferences for research on homeless veterans. *Community Mental Health Journal*, 35(3), 273–80.

Edwards, R. D. (1999) The good soldier. *The Sunday Times, Books*, 23 May, 1–2.

Finn, A. and Louviere, J. J. (1992) Determining the appropriate response to evidence of public concern – the case of food safety. *Journal of Public Policy and Marketing*, 11(2), 12–25.

Fise, M. E. R. (1992) Indoor air quality: a consumer protection issue. *Otolaryngology and Head and Neck Surgery*, 106(6), 665–8.

Graham, H. (1993) *When Life's a Drag: Women, Smoking and Disadvantage.* London: Department of Health.

Hanley, B., Truesdale, A., King, A., Elbourne, D. and Chalmers, I. (2001) Involving consumers in designing, conducting and interpreting randomized controlled trials. *British Medical Journal*, 322: 519–23.

Hannah, L., Rakotosamimanana, B., Ganzhorn, J. *et al.* (1998) Participatory planning, scientific priorities, and landscape conservation in Madagascar. *Environmental Conservation*, 25(1), 30–6.

Jones, T. (1985) *Chaucer's Knight: The Portrait of a Medieval Mercenary.* London: Methuen.

Lumley, J. (1991) Stopping smoking – again. *British Journal of Obstetrics and Gynaecology*, 98, 847–9.

Lumley, J. (1995) Strategies for reducing smoking in pregnancy. In the *Cochrane Pregnancy and Childbirth Database*, Issue 1. Oxford: Update Software.

Lumley, J., Oliver, S. and Waters, E. (1998) Smoking cessation programs implemented during pregnancy. In *The Cochrane Library*, Issue 3. Oxford: Update Software.

Maternity Alliance and NCH Action for Sick Children (1995) *Poor Expectations. Poverty and Undernourishment in Pregnancy: Summary.* London: Maternity Alliance and NCH.

Mills, B. F. and Karanja, D. D. (1997) Processes and methods for research programme priority setting: the experience of the Kenya Agricultural Research Institute Wheat Programme. *Food Policy*, 22(1), 63–79.

Minkes, J., Townsley, R., Weston, C. and Williams, C. (1995) Having a voice: involving people with learning difficulties in research. *British Journal of Learning Disabilities*, 23(3), 94–7.

Minkler, M. (1989) Health education, health promotion and the open society: an historical perspective. *Health Education Quarterly*, 16(1), 17–30.

Naisbitt, J. (1982) *Megatrends: Ten New Directions Transforming Our Lives.* New York: Warner Books.

Parkinson, D., Bromet, E. J. and Dew, M. A. (1989) Effectiveness of the United Steel Workers of America Coke Oven Intervention Program. *Journal of Occupational Medicine*, 31(5), 464–72.

Peersman, G. (1999) The 'targets' of health promotion. In S. Hood, B. Mayall and S. Oliver (eds) *Critical Issues in Social Research: Power and Prejudice.* Buckingham: Open University Press.

Phillimore, P. and Moffatt, S. (1994) Discounted knowledge: local experience, environmental pollution and health. In J. Popay and G. Williams (eds) *Researching the People's Health.* London and New York: Routledge.

Reilly, T. (1999) *Cromwell: An Honourable Enemy.* Dingle, Ireland: Brandon Publishers.

Rice, C., Roberts, H., Smith, S. and Bryce, C. (1994) 'It's like teaching your child to swim in a pool of alligators': lay voices and professional research on child accidents. In J. Popay and G. Williams (eds) *Researching the People's Health.* London and New York: Routledge.

Robinson, E., Rumsey, N. and Partridge, J. (1996) An evaluation of the impact of social interaction skills training for facially disfigured people. *British Journal of Plastic Surgery*, 49, 281–9.

Save the Children (1995) *You're on your own: young people's research in leaving care. Keynotes*, 12 (September), 6.

Sillars, S. (1983) *Chaucer's Prologue*. Cambridge: National Extension College.

Social Services Inspectorate and Arthritis Care (1996) *Disability and Isolation: A Joint SSI/Arthritis Care Study of Isolated People with Arthritis*. London: SSI/ Arthritis Care.

UK Coalition of People Living with HIV and AIDS (1996) *Report on the Needs Assessment of People Living with HIV and AIDS in the London Boroughs of Waltham Forest and Redbridge*. Unpublished, London.

▶ **13**

▷ Looking to the future: policies and
opportunities for better health

▷ **Ann Oakley and Sandy Oliver**

> In our approach to better health, we want to break with the past. We
> want to move beyond the old arguments and tired debates which have
> characterised so much consideration of public health issues, including
> those who say that nothing can be done to improve the health of the
> poorest and those who say that individuals are solely to blame for their
> own ill health . . . We reject the polarity of these positions.
> (Department of Health 1999: paras 1.22–4)

These challenging words come from the latest in a series of UK government
health policy documents, the White Paper *Saving Lives*. Taken together,
these documents indicate a marked shift in government policy towards the
role and meaning of health promotion. This shift is one of the pointers to
the future we look at in this chapter. But the call that is to be found in the
pages of *Saving Lives* to abandon past positions and arguments also summarizes many of the main themes of this book.

In this book we have highlighted the unhelpful ways in which health
promotion practice has often been caught between an 'individual' and a
'systems' approach – seeing people as responsible for their own health or ill
health, or as victims of healthy or unhealthy communities and sets of material circumstances. These polarities do nothing to represent faithfully the
evidence either of epidemiological research (Acheson 1998) or the ways in
which people experience everyday life and health (Cornwell 1984); thus
they are also an unproductive context for developing and assessing evidence about the value of health promotion initiatives. Our central focus
in this book has been on this question of evidence. Evidence, as we use
the term, encapsulates not only what is reliably known in a 'scientific' or
'academic' sense about effective health promotion, but the experiences of
those at whom health promotion interventions are targeted.

The centrality of 'subjective' or 'qualitative' data and the importance of a range of methods to the whole enterprise of assessing health promotion effectiveness signals another of our key themes: the disappointingly repetitive and sterile arguments about methods engaged in by many health promotion researchers and practitioners. The point is not whether 'quantitative' or 'qualitative' methods are better, but what these terms signify about professional allegiances and postures, all of which helps to explain what the arguments are 'really' about. Most important of all, of course, is selecting methods which are appropriate for answering particular research questions. Health promotion as an area of practical and academic endeavour has suffered hugely from a mismatch between method and question. The most important questions historically about health promotion have been those about what works, but, as various earlier chapters have shown, practitioners and researchers have overwhelmingly been engaged in studies which have not been able to answer these questions. Such studies may have provided all sorts of other valuable data, but this has not helped policy makers to make informed and cost-effective decisions between competing approaches for promoting the public health.

One of the cardinal tenets of the health promotion and public health movement has been that 'an ounce of prevention is worth a pound of cure' (Leichter 1991: 85). Governments' interest in health promotion has been dominated by its revenue-saving potential (Minkler 1989). This is an area in which little sustained work has been done, and there are certainly those who argue that on existing evidence health promotion is an expensive approach to promoting the public health (Russell 1986). Current weaknesses in the health promotion evidence-base also make it very difficult for the public to decide what they should do to protect their health. A general scepticism about the ability of health promotion to deliver anything worthwhile is hardly surprising in view of the conflicting advice the industry has offered the public over the years. In 'A medical sociologist looks at health promotion', Marshall Becker offers the following example:

> We all know that regular exercise is recommended for reducing the risk of heart disease. Unfortunately, recent data have pointed up the many thousands of injuries and hazards related to exercise, and has linked high levels of exercise to infertility, damage to the immune system, cancer, and premature aging. What to do? Run too little and die too young of a coronary? Run too much and experience shin splints and knee surgery and die, without offspring, of some bizarre infection?
> (Becker 1993: 1)

And who decides how much is too little or too much? Such examples suggest that a stronger and more accessible evidence-base is an ethical imperative, and also the mark of a democratically healthy society. There is a need for an evidence base which draws on academic and lay expertise, qualitative and quantitative data and can weigh the value of different approaches to promoting public health.

Identifying a lack of reliable evidence drawing on adequate methodologies or addressing questions and incorporating values important to those most intimately affected by health promotion may be seen as unreasonably nihilistic. It is certainly the conclusion reached over the past few years in a large number of health promotion review reports (Oakley *et al.* 1996a; Peersman *et al.* 1998; Harden *et al.* 1999) and critiques of health services research (Oliver 1997, 1999; Oliver *et al.* 1997; Oliver and Needham 1997; Oliver and Oakley 2001), and it is one we arrive at many times over in this book. Research and evaluation evidence in health promotion is generally hard to find, and sifting through what is there often produces a thin yield of well designed studies capable of offering convincing conclusions about effectiveness. We hope that some of the practical pointers we have provided in this book will make it easier for people to locate the kinds of health promotion research they want to find, to be more critical and informed about evaluating this evidence and also to be more aware of the interests of various stakeholder communities. Many people who undertake reviews of health promotion research emerge from this process impressed by how much work there is still to be done. The contrast between systematic reviewing and the selective picture gained by traditional literature reviews is particularly striking – writing a narrative description or reviewing a non-random sample of the literature can be a highly effective way of substituting researchers' opinions for research findings. This may be good for an academic *curriculum vitae* and the Research Assessment Exercise, but it hardly helps to build the evidence-base for health promotion as a practical, real-world activity. From this point of view, the conclusion that we do not know as much as we thought we did is a positive beginning, rather than a dispiriting brake to enthusiasm. We view it in this light in thinking about the future in this chapter.

Of course, many policy choices do not, and should not, depend on evidence, and none should depend on evidence alone; they reflect citizens' rights and responsibilities, and the accountability of governments to behave in moral ways. But choices that need evidence are not just difficult to make in health promotion. The same caveats apply to many domains of social intervention. For example, social welfare, public policy, criminology and education have traditionally shared with health promotion a reluctance to submit claims of professional expertise to the hard test of reliable evidence (MacDonald 1997). These areas are different from health care, where researchers have for many years been more aware of the need to guard against bias in determining what works. The example of the Cochrane Collaboration is in many ways a troubling one for those whose concern is social interventions such as health promotion. In principle there is no reason why an accessible, electronic library of constantly updated effectiveness reviews should not be an attractive and important aim. But there are also under-standable worries about 'hierarchies' of evidence and about accepting in-appropriate methodological standards which may be insufficiently sensitive to the contexts in which social interventions are deployed. These concerns point to the challenge of adapting the organizational and methodological practices of the Cochrane Collaboration to fit the requirements of social intervention evaluation, which include the task of sifting through a much higher proportion of non-experimental studies.

Towards a scientific evaluation policy?

Most of this book describes the results of a programme of work carried out at the EPPI-Centre, the Social Science Research Unit (SSRU), University of London Institute of Education. The starting point of this work in the early 1990s was a desire to map the extent and nature of evaluation activity in the social intervention field. When the work started there was enormous resistance to it, including among funders, who considered it fruitless to ask such trivial or, alternatively, over-ambitious questions. One of our earliest commissioned reviews, funded by the Medical Research Council, was of behavioural interventions for preventing the spread of HIV/AIDS (Oakley *et al.* 1995). The impetus for this was the realization that in the absence of effective medical treatments, health promotion is tremendously important as a strategy for preventing further transmission of the disease. The results of the review were surprising. A mere 2 per cent of a large literature pro-vided any reliable evidence as to the effectiveness of HIV/AIDS education. This pointed to a very considerable waste of money and effort on the part of many governments and individuals in launching and recommending particular education initiatives. The MRC review led to a series of others with similar findings in the field of sexual health (Oakley and Fullerton 1994; Oakley *et al.* 1996b; Peersman *et al.* 1996). These remain an import-ant framework for current policy initiatives in sexual health and the pre-vention of unintended teenage pregnancy as one of the UK government's foremost health targets.

Perhaps the biggest area of resistance in conducting and disseminating these reviews has been to seeing that such work, while it may appear to be preoccupied with small methodological issues, is of enormous policy sig-nificance. People's lives are harmed everyday by interventions carried out with entirely beneficial aims. This applies not only to doctors who prescribe medical treatments with quite devastating unanticipated consequences, such as thalidomide (a sedative which deformed unborn babies) or diethylstil-boestrol (prescribed to prevent miscarriages but resulting in daughters developing vaginal cancer), in two of the most famous examples. It also applies to social workers, teachers, politicians, health promoters and others who advocate approaches favoured because of fashion, shared professional norms or a belief that they *must* be effective. It may be genuinely difficult to understand the policy implications of fine-tuned methodological work. A persuasive example from health care is the findings of *Effective Care in Pregnancy and Childbirth* (Chalmers *et al.* 1989), the forerunner of the Cochrane Collaboration, which were hailed by a House of Commons Health Committee in 1992 as having 'profoundly influenced' its deliberations. The Committee commented that, had this work been available 20 years earlier, some of the most undesirable developments in the maternity services might never have taken place (Health Committee 1992). The Department of Health subsequently sent complimentary copies to all district health authorities; the results of the reviews were also incorporated into training material for health professionals, were taken up and used by activist groups in the maternity care field (Stocking 1993) and outside the UK were used to inform the work of health care decision-making bodies and to form the basis of new practice guidelines for professional organizations (Cochrane Centre 1992). Encouragingly, this work included reviews of social interventions, including health education.

There are many signs that the traditional resistance to evidence-informed policy-making in the social intervention arena is now breaking down. Academics, researchers and policy makers in Europe and North America are forming coalitions of interest around the notion of evidence-informed policy and practice. In 1996, Adrian Smith, professor of statistics, in a presidential address to the Royal Statistical Society in London, argued that 'We are, through the media, as ordinary citizens, confronted daily with controversy and debate across a whole spectrum of public policy issues. But typically, we have no access to any form of a systematic "evidence base" – and therefore no means of participating in the debate in a mature and informed manner.' Smith concluded that what is needed is a 'quantal shift' in public policy debates (Smith 1996). In the same year, David Hargreaves, professor of education at Cambridge, caused much controversy in educational circles with his lecture to the Teacher Training Agency entitled 'Teaching as a research-based profession: possibilities and prospects'. Like Smith, Hargreaves used the example of medicine to suggest that teaching is not at the moment an activity based on research and that teachers need to get their house in order (Hargreaves 1996).

Meetings convened in London in 1999 and in Philadelphia in 2000 subsequently proposed the formation of an international movement for research synthesis in public policy. These have now stimulated the establishment of the Campbell Collaboration as an analogue of the Cochrane Collaboration devoted to assembling an evidence-base for social and educational interventions. The Campbell Collaboration's initial register, SPECTR – the Social, Psychological and Educational Controlled Trials Register – holds bibliographic details of some 11,000 controlled trials (SPECTR 1999).

Research funders are now more committed to the need for a cumulative knowledge-base, and so are more willing than they used to be to support reviews work. The Economic and Social Research Council has recently funded a very substantial initiative in this area, which consists of a national coordinating centre and a number of subcentres engaged in policy reviews. On the government front, a number of UK government departments, including the Department for Education and Employment (DfEE), the Home Office and the Treasury, have joined the Department of Health in displaying a commitment to establishing evidence-base resources. In early 2000 the DfEE funded SSRU to set up a centre for evidence-informed policy and practice in education. This is an exciting initiative, which will mean that many of the streams of work discussed in this book will now be extended from health promotion to mainstream education.

Research, evaluation and policy-making in health promotion are all likely to benefit from this paradigm shift towards a stronger scientific base. The future for taking forward many of the themes highlighted in this book therefore looks bright. A further encouraging feature is the international aspect of the new stress on evidence-informed policy and practice. The research and evaluation vision has all too often been narrowly focused on local contexts, thereby missing the possibility for cross-cultural translation of lessons learned.

Acheson and all that

A second significant influence on the future of health promotion is the renewed political emphasis on inequalities in health. The Acheson report of the *Independent Inquiry into Inequalities in Health* in 1998 came out strongly in favour of a socio-economic model of health and its inequalities. The following list, which is taken from the Acheson report, shows the layers of influence which affect individual health outcomes.

1 General socio-economic, cultural and environmental conditions.
2 Living and working conditions
   • agricultural and food production;
   • education;
   • work environment;
   • unemployment;
   • water and sanitation;
   • health care services;
   • housing.
3 Social and community networks.
4 Individual lifestyle factors.
5 Age, sex and constitutional factors.

Important influences on people's abilities to maintain health are their living and working conditions, food supplies and access to essential goods and services. Economic, cultural and environmental conditions present in society as a whole form a further layer of influence. The research task is to trace the links between social structure and health outcomes; for health promotion this means respecting social structure (the 'systems approach') as the theoretical basis for interventions targeted at either individuals or communities. It means taking on board environmental constraints on individuals' abilities to make health-enhancing decisions. The effects of poverty and social disadvantage are thus significant players in the arena of health promotion decision-making.

The epidemiological evidence informing the Acheson and other recent government reports is that of 'unacceptable inequalities in health' persisting in the UK, despite falls in average mortality over the past 50 years (Acheson Report 1998: xi). *Saving Lives* (para. 4.2) puts it quite unequivocally:

> Health inequality runs throughout life, from before birth through into old age. It exists between social classes, different areas of the country, between men and women, and between people from different ethnic backgrounds. But the story of health inequality is clear: the poorer you are, the more likely you are to be ill and to die younger. That is true for almost every health problem.

For many measures of health, these inequalities have either remained the same or widened over past decades. The policy implications are therefore that improving health and reducing health inequalities ought to be integrated aims. What holds for the UK is also true more globally; the World Bank has estimated that poor material environments account for some 30 per cent of the global burden of disease (World Bank 1993). Cross-national comparisons in Organization for Economic Cooperation and Development countries also suggest a relationship between disparities in income distribution and life expectancy; the healthier countries are the ones with the smallest income inequalities (Wilkinson 1992).

Less polarization and more integration

An impressive initiative to tackle inequalities in Britain is the establishment of 'Health Action Zones', which aim to develop and implement a health strategy that cuts inequalities and delivers measurable improvements in public health and health outcomes, and the quality of treatment and care. The Health Action Zone approach is underpinned by seven principles of achieving equity, engaging communities, working in partnership, engaging frontline staff, taking an evidence-based approach, developing a person-centred approach to service delivery and taking a whole systems approach.

These principles jettison old polarities of research and practice, professional and lay, and individual and 'system', but they do not necessary fully integrate these different perspectives.

Another advance in rejecting polarities is the concept of 'needs-led' research programmes. Before the launch of the NHS Research and Development Strategy in 1991 there had been no systematic attempt to relate important health issues to the national effort in medical research. 'Innovation in medical research [had] been driven largely by the intrinsic interests of disease processes to clinicians and scientists' (Peckham 1991). Since then health practitioners in both treatment and health promotion services have been engaged in a series of formal research agenda setting exercises for cancer, asthma, etc. (NHS Executive 1994, 1995a, b; NHS Management Executive 1994).

An even more inclusive policy is involving service users in research. This has had particular impetus from the NHS Executive since 1996 through its standing committee, Consumers in NHS Research. Consumers in NHS Research aims to ensure that consumer involvement in research and development in the NHS improves the way that research is prioritized, commissioned, undertaken and disseminated. Its strategic objectives are: to develop strategic alliances with key groups in order to promote greater consumer involvement in health research; to empower consumers to become more involved in research and development in the NHS; and to monitor and evaluate the effects of consumer involvement in NHS research and development.

An obvious question is: to what extent do consumer contributions to health research repeat, extend, complement or conflict with those of health professionals and professional researchers? Consumer activities often focus particularly on the social and emotional aspects of research: patient information and support for health care and for research, and social and emotional aspects of ill health and health care. When consumers and professionals work together, they bring different skills to the research. Professionals may bring a formality and credibility appropriate to professional audiences and access to professional journals, while consumers gain access and improve recruitment because of their credibility among their peers. There are examples of professionals bringing technical skills to consumer research agendas. For instance, when the Hodgkin's Disease and Lymphoma Association asked its members and recent enquirers about their concerns about delays in referrals, patients' experience of presenting symptoms and lack of information and support, their questionnaire was designed with the help of the association's medical advisors, representatives of the Royal College of General Practitioners and the Cancer Research Campaign Communication and Counselling Centre.

Managerial roles may be undertaken by consumers recruiting researchers for 'in-house' projects. The National Cancer Alliance approached researchers when it wished to find out to what extent cancer services take account of patients', families' and carers' views (National Cancer Alliance 1996). Alternatively, professionals may provide the management skills and draw on consumers for advice, access to those being researched and data collection. Another project was the MAIN (Multisite randomized controlled trial of Alternative treatments for flat or Inverted Nipples) trial. This coincided with the research agenda of the National Childbirth Trust, which provided volunteer networks and breastfeeding counsellors, and this increased trial recruitment, which was otherwise proving a problem (Renfrew and McCandlish 1992; MAIN Trial Collaborative Group 1994).

These examples reflect a mosaic of activities which have flourished within the voluntary sector because people have invested their time or their money in response to their perception of services or research as inadequate in quality or quantity. Formally integrating individuals and groups from outside the NHS potentially harnesses their energy, experiences and creativity.

Where does this leave health promotion? First of all, it suggests new alliances: health promotion *and* public health *and* the public. The old public health movement is re-emerging in a new form, with a consequent thinning of the boundaries between it and much of what has customarily been defined as health promotion. The link with public health represents an even greater move for health promotion away from the old-style health education, which began to go out of vogue in the 1970s with the growing realization that offering information rarely in itself empowers people to behave in healthier ways.

The new emphasis on public health also highlights awkward questions about who has benefited most from health promotion activity. Indeed, the impact of much health promotion may have been to widen inequality, because the better off have been more receptive and able to take note of health promotion messages. One example is an intervention in Northern England designed to improve uptake of immunization among children, which found that inequalities between deprived and affluent areas persisted or even widened when coverage increased substantially (Reading *et al.* 1994). A systematic review of interventions aimed at reducing inequalities in health reported on 94 studies and 21 reviews, which amounted to a general lack of good evidence about effective approaches, particularly in the UK (Arblaster *et al.* 1996). The results of this review were hailed as 'disappointing' in the report *Variations in Health: What Can the Department of Health and the NHS Do?* by the Chief Medical Officer's Health of the Nation Working Group (Variations Sub-Group 1995).

The implications of this newly focused thinking about health promotion and public health include the UK government's decision to change the Health Education Authority into the Health Development Agency, whose key functions will include maintaining a database of the evidence for public health and health improvement. A second major implication is the need for a strong and high-quality academic base to support research. A key feature of this infrastructure will be the collation of research information, which at the moment is held and managed by different agencies (*Saving Lives* paras 11.38 and 11.27). Following the success of government publishing on the Internet and in line with the objectives of the Citizens' Charter and Open Government, this information will be accessible to practitioners, researchers and the public alike. For evidence also to be open to debate, whether it is drawn from literature reviews, individuals studies, audits or opinion, it must include 'a clear and transparent account of how it was collated, which sources of information have been consulted, who was involved in the process of collating the evidence, how the work was funded, and a full disclosure of any analysis and findings.' (Gillies 1999). For debate to ensue, the time and the skills to consider evidence need to be spread among policy makers, practitioners and the public. Methods and resources to facilitate this are already available (Milne and Oliver 1996; Oliver *et al.* 1996; Parkes *et al.* 2000; Oliver and Oakley 2001; for critical appraisal skills see Chapter 11). Greater transparency and more informed debate, drawing on the experience of public health, health promotion and people's daily lives, will not only call decision-makers to account, but may lead to more real solutions to pressing problems.

References

Acheson Report (1998) *Independent Inquiry into Inequalities in Health*. London: HMSO.

Arblaster, L., Lambert, M., Entwhistle, V. *et al.* (1996) A systematic review of the effectiveness of health service interventions aimed at reducing inequalities in health. *Journal of Health Services Research and Policy*, 1(2), 93–103.

Becker, M. H. (1993) A medical sociologist looks at health promotion, *Journal of Health and Social Behavior*, 34, 1–6.

Chalmers, I., Enkin, M. and Kierse, M. J. N. C. (eds) (1989) *Effective Care in Pregnancy and Childbirth*. Oxford: Oxford University Press.

Cochrane Centre (1992) *Brochure*. Oxford: Cochrane Centre.

Cornwell, J. (1984) *Hard-earned Lives*. London: Tavistock.

Department of Health (1999) *Saving Lives: Our Healthier Nation*. London: HMSO.

Dahlgren, G. and Whitehead, M. (1991) *Policies and Strategies to Promote Social Equity in Health*. Stockholm: Institute of Futures Studies.

Gillies, P. (1999) *Evidence Base 2000: Evidence into Practice*. London: Health Education Authority.

Harden, A., Peersman, G., Oliver, S., Mauthuner, M. and Oakley, A. (1999) A systematic review of the effectiveness of health promotion interventions in the workplace. *Occupational Medicine*, 49, 1–9.

Hargreaves, D. H. (1996) Teaching as a research-based profession: possibilities and prospects. Teaching Training Agency Annual Lecture.

Health Committee (1992) *Second Report, Session 1991–2. Maternity Services*. London: HMSO.

Leichter, H. M. (1991) *Free to Be Foolish: Politics and Health Promotion in the United States and Great Britain*. Princeton, NJ: Princeton University Press.

MacDonald, G. (1997) Social work: beyond control? In A. Maynard and I. Chalmers (eds) *Effectiveness and Efficiency: Some Non-random Reflections on Health Services*. London: BMJ Publishing.

MAIN Trial Collaborative Group (1994) Preparing for breastfeeding: treatment of inverted and non-protractile nipples in pregnancy. *Midwifery*, 10, 200–14.

Milne, R. and Oliver, S. (1996) Evidence-based consumer health information: developing teaching in critical appraisal skills. *International Journal for Quality in Health Care*, 8(5), 439–45.

Minkler, M. (1989) Health education, health promotion and the open society: an historical perspective. *Health Education Quarterly*, 16(1), 17–30.

National Cancer Alliance (1996) *Patient-centred Cancer Services? What Patients Say*. Oxford: National Cancer Alliance.

NHS Executive (1994) *R&D Priorities in Cancer. Report to the NHS Central Research and Development Committee*. Leeds: Department of Health.

NHS Executive (1995a) *Improving the Health of Mothers and Children: NHS Priorities for Research and Development*. Leeds: Department of Health.

NHS Executive (1995b) *Methods to Promote the Implementation of Research Findings in the NHS. Priorities for Evaluation*. Leeds: Department of Health.

NHS Management Executive (1994) *R&D Priorities in Relation to the Interface between Primary and Secondary Care. Report to the NHS Central Research and Development Committee*. Leeds: NHS Management Executive.

Oakley, A., France-Dawson, M., Fullerton, D. *et al.* (1996a) Preventing falls and subsequent injury in older people. *Effective Health Care Bulletin*, 2, 4.

Oakley, A. and Fullerton, D. (1994) *Risk, Knowledge and Behaviour: HIV/AIDS Education Programmes and Young People*. London: Social Science Research Unit.

Oakley, A., Fullerton, D. and Holland, J. (1995) Behavioural interventions for HIV/AIDS prevention. *AIDS*, 9, 479–86.

Oakley, A., Oliver, S., Peersman, G. and Mauthner, M. (1996b) *Review of effectiveness of Health Promotion Interventions for Men who Have Sex with Men*. London: EPI-Centre, Social Science Research Unit.

Oliver, S. (1997) Exploring lay perspectives on questions of effectiveness. In A. Maynard and I. Chalmers (eds) *Effectiveness and Efficiency: Some Non-random Reflections on Health Services*. London: BMJ Publishing.

Oliver, S. (1999) Users of health services: following their agenda. In S. Hood, B. Mayall and S. Oliver (eds) *Critical Issues in Social Research: Power and Prejudice*. Buckingham: Open University Press.

Oliver, S., Crowe, S. and Needham, G. (1997) Is routine amniotomy good for childbearing women and their babies? What can we learn from a randomised controlled trial? *British Journal of Midwifery*, 5(4), 228–30.

Oliver, S. and Needham, G. (1997) Continuity of carer: what can we learn from a Cochrane review? *British Journal of Midwifery*, 5(5), 292–5.

Oliver, S., Nicholas, A. and Oakley, A. (1996) *Promoting Health after Sifting the Evidence (PHASE) Workshop Report*. London: EPI-Centre.

Oliver, S. and Oakley, A. (2001) The labouring mother. In G. Chamberlain and P. Steer (eds) *Turnbull's Obstetrics*, 3rd edn. London: Harcourt Brace.

Parkes, J., Deeks, J., Milne, R. and Hyde, C. (2000) Teaching critical appraisal skills in health care settings (protocol for a Cochrane Review). In *The Cochrane Library*, Issue 2. Oxford: Update Software.

Peckham, M. (1991) Research and development for the National Health Service. *Lancet*, 367–71.

Peersman, G., Harden, A. and Oliver, S. (1998) *Effectiveness of Health Promotion Interventions in the Workplace: A Review*. London: Health Education Authority.

Peersman, G., Oakley, A., Oliver, S. and Thomas, J. (1996) *Review of Effectiveness of Sexual Health Promotion Interventions for Young People*. London: EPI-Centre, Social Science Research Unit.

Reading, R., Colver, A., Openshaw, S. and Jarvis S. (1994) Do interventions that improve immunisation uptake also reduce social inequalities in uptake? *British Medical Journal*, 308, 1142–4.

Renfrew, M. J. and McCandlish, R. (1992) With women: new steps in research in midwifery. In H. Roberts (eds) *Women's Health Matters*. London: Routledge.

Russell, L. (1986) *Is Prevention Better than Cure?* Washington, DC: The Brookings Institution.

Smith, A. (1996) Presidential address to the Royal Statistical Society, London.

SPECTR (1999) *Social, Psychological and Educational Controlled Trials Register*. Oxford: Update Software.

Stocking, B. (1993) Implementing the findings of Effective Care in Pregnancy and Childbirth in the United Kingdom. *Milbank Quarterly*, 71(3), 497–521.

Variations Sub-Group (1995) *Variations in Health: What Can the Department of Health and the NHS Do?* London: HMSO.

Wilkinson, R. (1992) Income distribution and life expectancy. *British Medical Journal*, 304, 165–8.

World Bank (1993) *World Development Report 1993: Investing in Health*. Washington, DC: World Bank.

▷ Index